The Essential Guide for Living Well with Diabetes

The Essential Guide for Living Well with Diabetes

Simple ways to avoid Diabetes (Reduce the Carbs, Shed Weight, and Feel Great Now!)

GUIDELINE

Wellington 365

Table of Contents

Preface

In this century a lot is said about the non-communicable disease and healthy living unlike back in the 90s when there was a lot about infectious diseases and injuries that were curable now, in this era it's about non – communicable diseases that are caused by certain lifestyle activities and are diet-related.

This book contains all the information you need to prevent yourself from any of the non-communicable diseases, it provides you with the best sources of information to help you make an informed decision about your life and how to live a healthy lifestyle to prevent all forms of non-communicable diseases with this book you take charge of your health and lifestyle because non-communicable diseases are not curable but can be managed.

About the Author

Wellington 365 is an American nutritionist with a piece of in-depth knowledge about nutrition. He has an MPhil in nutrition and worked with people with all forms of non-communicable disease to achieve good and healthy well-being, which is my goal because of my love and passion for nutrition and healthy living.

Reading this book will help you identify ways to preclude diabetes and all forms of non-communicable diseases it contains relevant and particle information on nutrition and healthy living.

“We spend trillions of dollars to Cure or Manage a disease when prevention of those diseases is a simple change of Diet”

Introduction

Good nutrition is a principal aspect of healthy living, but healthy eating and avoiding junk foods can be challenging, unlike in the early ages when health issues were mostly infectious diseases and injuries now the 21st century due to the significance of public health, medical advancement, and economic development communicable disease are no longer of public health concern but Chronic Diseases are also known as non-communicable diseases (NCDs).

Non-communicable diseases (NCDs) are the leading causes of death and the central issue in contemporary and future public health globally. Noncommunicable diseases (NCDs) account for 41 million annual fatalities or 71% of all fatalities worldwide. Currently, NCD deaths are more prevalent among the ages of 30 and 69 years, as more than 15 million people per year die from an NCD with 85% of these "premature" deaths in low- and middle-income nations. The majority of NCD deaths, or 17.9 million people per year, are caused by cardiovascular diseases, followed by cancers (9.3 million), respiratory illnesses (4.1 million), and diabetes (1.5 million).

It's great you found this book because this book contains all the relevant information on how to prevent you and your family from diabetes and other forms of non-communicable diseases, this book also provides in-depth knowledge on the nutritional advances, health, recent evidence, and practical information which will inform your decision on healthy living to prevent all forms of non-communicable disease.

Most health professionals believed that once you developed diabetes, you were stuck with it—and could anticipate one health issue after another, from worsening eyesight and nerve symptoms to heart and kidney problems. But this simply is not true. The research has shown that it is often possible to improve insulin sensitivity and tackle type 2 diabetes by following my step-by-step plan, which includes a healthful vegan diet with plenty of recipes to get started, an exercise guide, advice about taking supplements and tracking progress, and troubleshooting tips.

CHAPTER 1

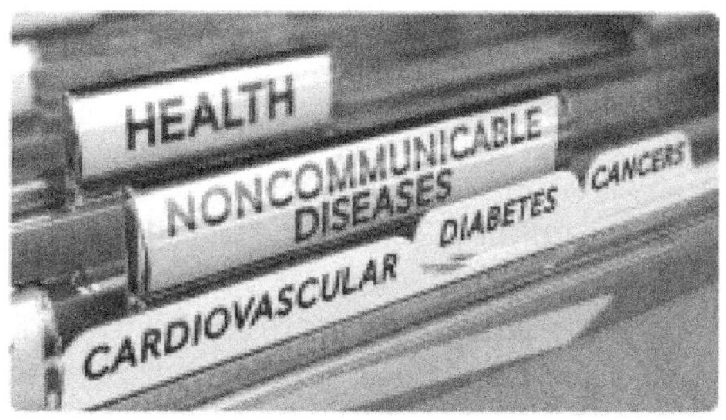

What are Non- communicable Diseases (NCDs)?

"Non-communicable diseases" is the umbrella term for diseases that are not passed from person to person, they are the single biggest factor dominating the health and longevity of modern humans.

Chronic diseases sometimes referred to as non-communicable diseases (NCDs), are conditions that develop over an extended period because of a combination of genetic, physiological, environmental, and behavioral variables. The four primary categories of NCD include diabetes, cancer, chronic respiratory diseases like chronic obstructive pulmonary disease and asthma, and cardiovascular disorders like heart attacks and strokes. With NCDs, early detection is key unlike other communicable diseases NCDs can only be managed and not cured therefore palliative care is the component of the response.

Prevalence of Non-Communicable Diseases

The burden of NCDs worldwide is still too high. Out of the 57 million deaths worldwide in 2016, NCDs caused 41 million (71%) of them, and 15 million deaths were premature (30 to 70 years). In low- and middle-income nations, where 78% of all NCD fatalities and 85% of premature deaths occurred, the burden is greatest. Additionally, about 800,000 deaths in 2016 were caused by suicide. A slight relative decrease of 6% from 2010 has reduced the risk of dying too soon from one of the four major NCDs to 18% in 2016. 9.6 million premature deaths might be prevented by 2025. One of the biggest health challenges of the twenty-first century is the prevalence of non-communicable diseases (NCDs), which are the leading cause of death worldwide. A political statement to boost international and national efforts to prevent and control NCDs was made in September 2011 at the United Nations General Assembly in New York. WHO was granted a leadership position as part of the declaration, and as a result, the WHO Global Action Plan for the Prevention and Control of NCDs 2013-2020 (Global NCD Action Plan) was created and approved by the World Health Assembly in 2013.

Risk factors of NCDs

Avoidable risk factors are largely to blame for the rise in NCDs. The four primary behavioral risk factors of NCD tobacco use, harmful alcohol use, physical inactivity, and poor diet are causally related to the four major NCDs (cardiovascular disease, cancer, chronic respiratory illness, and diabetes). Four major metabolic/physiological alterations are the result of these behaviors: elevated blood pressure, overweight/obesity, elevated blood glucose, and elevated blood lipids. A significant risk factor is also environmental air pollution.

Environmental and Physiological influence on the development of non-communicable diseases

The early years of life are when environmental factors like the mother's food, body composition, and stress exposure have an impact on the development of her fetus and baby, determining how they will react to future environmental difficulties like an obesogenic lifestyle. Through the sperm, the paternal lifestyle can potentially have an impact on development. By facilitating a quick phenotypic response to an environmental change, such paternal impacts may confer a fitness advantage. When the cues that the developing embryo and fetus pick up on are inaccurate, such as when the mother's diet is unbalanced or when there is a nutritional transition between generations due to migration or rapid economic growth, the offspring's responses to subsequent environmental challenges are mismatched, which increases the risk of NCD, Although undernutrition is still a major issue in developing countries, overnutrition and undernutrition have negative effects in both developing and industrialized civilizations with a chance that results can be passed down across several generations. The effects have a wide range of life-course effects, such as behavioral issues, impaired cognition, osteoporosis, sarcopenia, and various allergy disorders. The underlying mechanisms have now been identified through epidemiological, clinical, and basic scientific research, many of which include epigenetic processes. These can therefore act as early warning signs of future increased risk of non-communicable disease.

A sedentary lifestyle and the consumption of unhealthy foods such as a high-fat diet, sugar-sweetened beverages, and increased screen time also predispose an individual to NCDs .

Genetic factors that influence the development of non-communicable diseases

The presence of one or more genetic mutations or a combination of alleles can increase the risk non- communicable disease however research is still ongoing on the relationship between genetic factors and the susceptibility to non-communicable disease, with cancers such as breast and ovarian cancers research has established the genetic influence through genotyping which is used to determine the severity, recurrences and to inform treatment for breast and ovarian cancers. In diabetes gene variant encoding the transcription factor of 7(TCF7L2) is said to increase the risk of diabetes as compared to the non-variant carrier however this genome has been used in the pharmaceutical and clinical practices to improve the management of diabetes (Florez et al., 2006; Meigs et al., 2008).

Behavioral factors that influence the development of non-communicable disease

The risk of NCDs is increased by several modifiable behaviors, including smoking, being physically inactive, unhealthy eating habits, and abusing alcohol. According to the World Health Organization, over 7.2 million people die from tobacco-related causes each year, and that number is expected to rise significantly in the coming years (including deaths brought on by exposure to passive smoking) and 4.1 million fatalities each year from overconsumption of salt and sodium with more than half of the 3.3 million deaths per year linked to alcohol use are caused by NCDs, such as cancer. Alcohol abuse is a significant contributor to early mortality and disability worldwide and is known to increase the chance of developing heart disease, cancer, liver disease, a variety of mental and behavioral disorders, other noncommunicable diseases, and communicable infections (Wood et al., 2021).

Harmful Alcohol and Tobacco use

Alcohol-related harm is influenced by both overall alcohol consumption and drinking habits, such as binge drinking on occasion. In 2010, the World Health Assembly supported a global strategy to minimize alcohol abuse that identified areas for multisectoral action to lessen the burden of diseases linked to alcohol consumption. One of the main global risk factors for illness and mortality from major NCDs is presently tobacco use, which includes both smoking and using smokeless tobacco. These negative health effects are brought on not just by smoking directly, but also by second-hand smoke exposure among non-smokers. Tobacco use poses a serious hazard to one's health.

Reduce Physical inactivity

The increasing severity of NCDs is also fuelled by physical inactivity. Comparing those who engage in at least 30 minutes of moderate-intensity physical exercise most days of the week to people who are not physically active enough have a higher chance of developing any of the NCDs.

Additionally, exercise reduces the risk of heart attack, high blood pressure, and depression. At the Sixty-sixth World Health Assembly in 2013, Member States agreed on a global objective of a 10% decrease in levels of physical inactivity by 2025 in recognition of the close ties between physical exercise and both physical and mental health. A worldwide action plan to promote physical activity was introduced by WHO in 2018 to update countries' instructions and promote a framework of practical and successful policy initiatives to enhance physical activity at all levels of society as lack of physical inactivity is account for 1.6 million deaths each year

Salt intake

A salt-rich diet raises blood pressure and raises the chance of developing heart disease and stroke. The recommended daily consumption of sodium is less than 2 grams of sodium or 5 grams of salt to lower the risk. The average population's salt intake is one of the global NCD targets, and it is expected to decrease by 30% relative by 2025.

Estimates from 2010 reveal that people worldwide consume an average of 9-12 grams of salt per day, which is twice the recommended daily dose, even though data on the mean population intake of sodium is currently not generally available.

People at risk of non-communicable diseases

NCDs affect all age groups, geographical areas, and nations, even though more than 15 million of all fatalities attributable to NCDs occur in people between the ages of 30 and 69 years, this disease was usually associated with the elderly but now 85% of these "premature" deaths are thought to take place in low- and middle-income nations. Children, adults, and seniors are all susceptible to the risk factors for NCDs, including poor diets, inactivity, exposure to tobacco use, and harmful alcohol use. NCDs are driven by the nutrition transition in developing countries which is the dietary shift from the consumption of local staple foods to processed foods coupled with a sedentary lifestyle, rapid unplanned urbanization, globalization of unhealthy lifestyles, and population aging. Unhealthy diets and a lack of physical activity may result in elevated blood pressure, increased blood glucose, elevated blood lipids, and obesity. These are called metabolic risk factors that can lead to cardiovascular disease, the leading NCD in terms of premature deaths, it's not a disease of affluence but poses an increasing threat to global health and the economies of both developed and developing countries, where they have overtaking communicable diseases.

What are metabolic risk factors?

These are a group of risk factors that are particularly associated with cardiovascular disease or non-communicable disease, these risk factors increase your likelihood of diabetes, heart disease, stroke, or all three significantly increased by metabolic syndrome. Experts are unsure about the exact cause of metabolic risk factors. There are several variables related to the risk factors examples of these metabolic risk factors include.

Elevated blood pressure

Hypertension, another name for high blood pressure, is elevated blood pressure. Depending on your activity, your blood pressure changes throughout the day. A diagnosis of high blood pressure may be made if blood pressure readings are frequently higher than normal. A person is diagnosed with high blood pressure if the systolic pressure reads 130 mm/Hg and above while the diastolic pressure is 90 mm/Hg and above. Your risk of developing additional health issues, such as heart disease, a heart attack, and stroke, increases as your blood pressure levels rise.

A table of the classification of high blood pressure

ACC/AHA 2017 HYPERTENSION GUIDELINES (13TH NOV 2017)
New Classification for Hypertension

CATEGORY	SYSTOLIC BP (MM HG)		DIASTOLIC BP (MM HG)	COMPARISON WITH JNC 7
NORMAL	<120	AND	<80	--
ELEVATED BP	120-129	AND	<80	*Was classified as Pre-hypertension under JNC7*
STAGE 1	130-139	OR	80-89	
STAGE 2	≥ 140	OR	≥ 90	*SBP of 140-159 OR DBP of 90-99 mm Hg was classified as Stage 1 under JNC7*
HYPERTENSIVE CRISIS	≥ 180	OR	≥ 120	--

Compiled by PlexusMD

Causes and effects of high blood pressure

Elevated blood pressure is the primary metabolic risk factor, and is responsible for 19% of fatalities worldwide). Most often, high blood pressure has no symptoms or warning indications, and many people are unaware they have it. The only method to determine whether you have high blood pressure is to measure it. Usually, high blood pressure comes on gradually. Unhealthy lifestyle activities, such as low physical activity, Obesity, and certain medical problems like diabetes might raise one's risk of acquiring high blood pressure. Pregnancy can also cause high blood pressure which is known as pregnancy-induced hypertension is resolved after delivery but predisposes the mother to hypertension. High blood pressure can harm your health in numerous ways that can cause severe damage to your heart, brain, kidneys, and eyes. but the good news is that managing your blood pressure can usually reduce your chance of developing major health issues and this book is to provide you with all the information you need for healthy living (High Blood Pressure Symptoms and Causes | Cdc.Gov, n.d.).

High blood pressure can result in making your arteries less elastic, and high blood pressure can harm them, which reduces the flow of blood and oxygen to your heart and increases the risk of heart disease. Additionally, the reduced blood supply to the heart can result in angina or chest pain.

A heart attack occurs when your heart's blood supply is cut off and the heart muscle starts to die from a lack of oxygen. The more time the blood flow is restricted, the more harm the heart sustains.

Heart failure is a disorder where the heart is unable to adequately pump blood and oxygen to the body's other organs.

High blood pressure can rupture or become blocked in the arteries that carry blood and oxygen to the brain, which can result in a stroke. During a stroke, brain cells perish because they do not receive enough oxygen. Serious impairments in speech, movement, and other everyday activities can result after a stroke. An additional fatality is a stroke. Also, high blood pressure is associated with dementia and impaired cognitive performance later in life, particularly in midlife. High blood pressure can also result in chronic kidney disease.

Overweight/obesity

Overweight and obesity are abnormal or excessive fat accumulation that could harm one's health. Body mass index (BMI) is a simple measure of weight about height that is frequently used to categorize adults as overweight or obese. It is determined by dividing the individual's weight in kilograms by the square of his or her height in meters (kg/m2) weight is BMI greater than or equal to 25 and obesity is a BMI greater than or equal to 30. Since 1975, the global rate of obesity has nearly tripled as over 1.9 billion persons aged 18 and older were overweight in 2016 and 650 million of these people were obese. Being overweight or obese kills more people than being underweight in most obesity-endemic countries however obesity is preventable.

Causes and effects of obesity

Obesity and overweight are primarily caused by an imbalance in energy between calories consumed and calories burned. Globally, there has been a rise in the consumption of calorie-dense foods that are rich in fat and sugar as well as an increase in physical inactivity because of the changing modes of transportation, rising urbanization, and the sedentary nature of many occupations. The lack of supportive policies in areas including health, agriculture, transportation, urban planning, environment, food processing, distribution, marketing, and education often leads to environmental and sociological changes that affect dietary and physical activity habits.

The leading causes of death in 2012 were cardiovascular diseases (primarily heart disease and stroke), diabetes, musculoskeletal disorders (especially osteoarthritis, a severely disabling degenerative disease of the joints), and some cancers. BMI is a significant risk factor for these noncommunicable diseases. As BMI increases, the risk for these noncommunicable diseases also increases. Childhood obesity increases the risk of adulthood obesity, premature death, and disability. However, obese children also experience breathing issues, an increased risk of fractures, hypertension, early indicators of cardiovascular disease, insulin resistance, and psychological effects in addition to their increased future risks .

Symptoms of diabetes

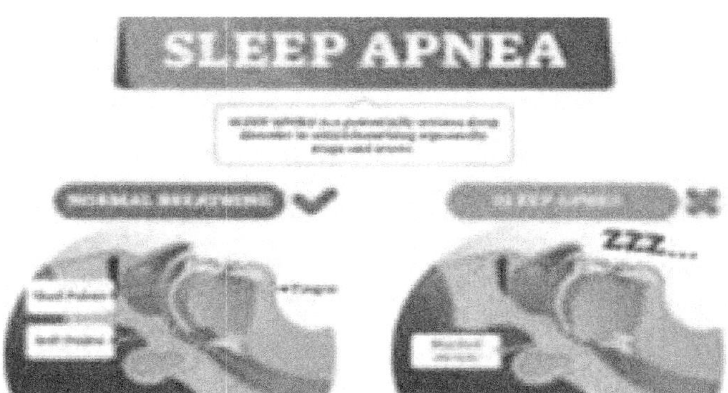

General symptoms

Diabetes symptoms are caused by rising blood sugar. The general symptoms of diabetes include:

- Nausea
- Excessive urination
- Intense hunger
- Intense thirst
- Numbness of limbs
- Reduced resistance to infections
- Blurred
- Weight loss
- Frequent urination
- Extreme fatigue

- Sores that don't heal

Specific symptoms in men

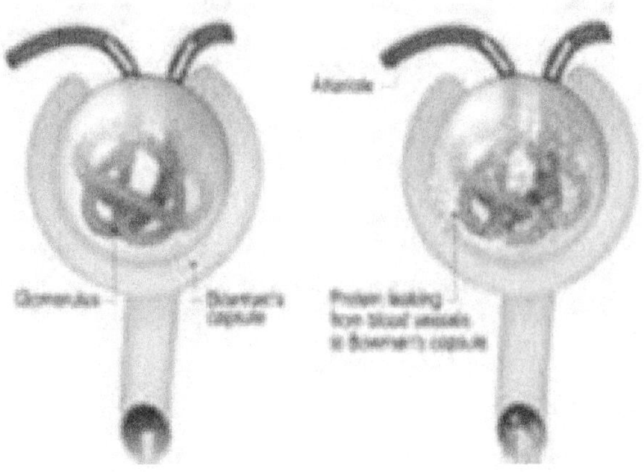

In addition to the general symptoms of diabetes, men with diabetes may have a decreased sex drive, erectile dysfunction (E.D.), and poor muscle strength due to high blood sugar level that has not been adequately controlled.

Specific symptoms in women

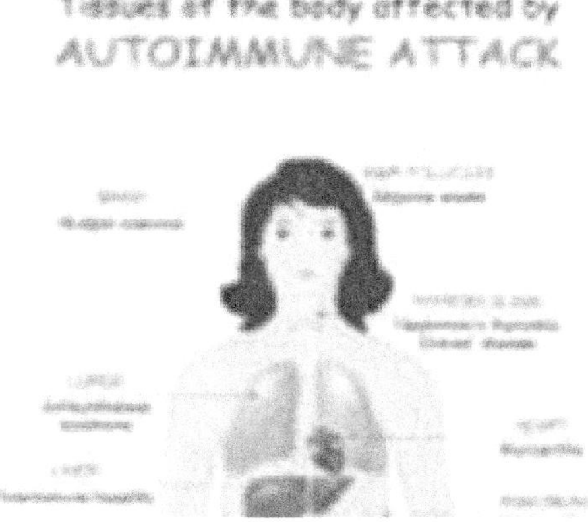

Urinary tract infections, yeast infections, dry, itchy skin, and an odorous vagina can also be signs of diabetes in women. Vaginal discharges are distinct from regular vaginal discharge and might occasionally be present in conjunction with a vaginal infection.

What causes diabetic nerve damage

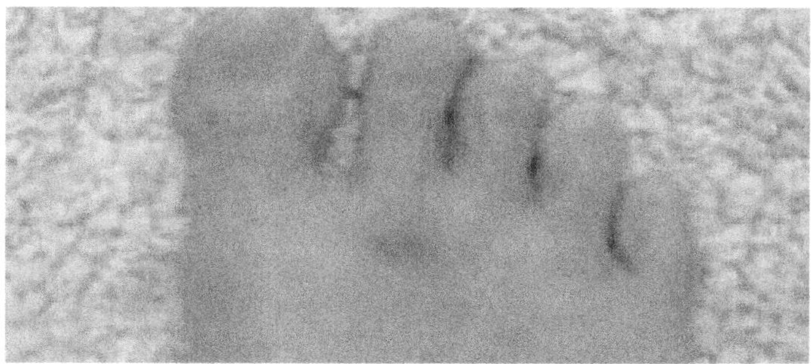

High blood sugar level that has existed for an extended period is the leading cause of damage to nerve endings. Why and how high blood sugar levels cause nerve damage is yet not known. One possible reason is the intricate interplay between the blood vessels and nerves, according to NIDDK.

Other factors perceived to be responsible include high blood pressure, high cholesterol levels, and nerve inflammation. Diabetic peripheral neuropathy appears first in the feet and legs and later in the arms .

Feeling numbness

Numbness is a common symptom of diabetic peripheral neuropathy. A diabetic patient suffering from peripheral neuropathy may sometimes be unable to feel that they are walking while walking. There may also be a tingling and burning sensation in the hands and feet or a feeling of wearing a sock while no socks are worn on any of the feet. That is why such an individual may have cut on the feet or arm without feeling it. Such injury also makes it difficult to heal and may lead to amputation of such a limb. Patients should always wear protective footwear and be careful not to sustain avoidable physical injuries.

Where is diabetes more prevalent?

Four out of five people in the world with diabetes now live in low- and middle-income countries (LMIC), and the incidence of diabetes is increasing in poorer communities. Diabetes increases susceptibility to infection and worsens outcomes for some of the world's major infectious diseases, such as tuberculosis, melioidosis, and dengue. However, the relationship between diabetes and many neglected tropical diseases is yet to be adequately quantified. There is some evidence that chronic viral infections such as hepatitis B and HIV may predispose an individual to the development of type 2 diabetes by chronic inflammatory and immune metabolic mechanisms. Helminth infections such as schistosomiasis may be protective against the development of diabetes. This finding opens up new territory for discovering novel therapeutics for the prevention and treatment of diabetes.

To develop vaccines and treatments for the growing population of people with diabetes who are at risk of infection, as well as to pay more attention to research works as well as public health interventions and policy, it is necessary to have a better understanding of the impact of diabetes on risksand outcomes for infections causing significant diseases in LMIC. I was able to discuss the prevalence of diabetes today around the world, the evidence for interactions between diabetes and infection, the immune mechanisms underlying the interaction, and potential interventions to fight the co-infection of diabetes and other on-diabetic infections like dengue, melioidosis, tropical, and tuberculosis.

About 336 million people with diabetes are now living in low and middle-income countries (LMIC). Types 1 and 2 diabetes increase susceptibility to infection and worsen the outcomes for diseases such as tuberculosis (T.B.). Current international treatment guidelines for diabetes are based on research conducted in high-income countries focused on preventing adverse cardiovascular diseases and early death. There is no empirical evidence to base guidelines for people living in LMIC, where there is an increased incidence of infectious diseases compared with high-income countries.

Unique symptoms of type1 diabetes can include

- Extreme hunger
- Increased thirst
- Deistic weight loss
- Frequent urination
- Blurry vision
- Tiredness

- Occasional mood changes

Hyperglycaemia (high blood glucose levels)

The medical term for high blood sugar is hyperglycemia. When the body doesn't produce enough insulin or uses it improperly, high blood sugar results.

THE GLUCOSE LEVEL

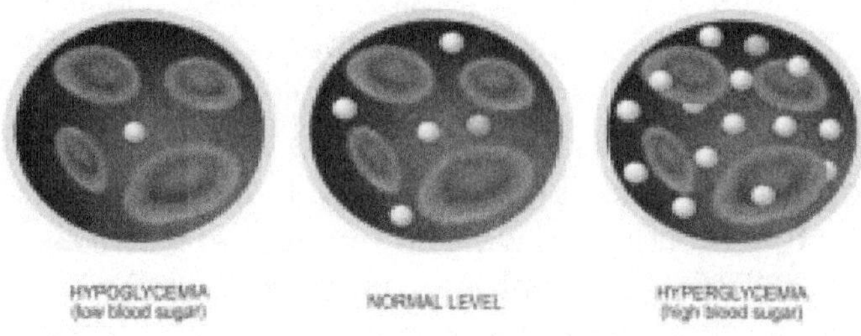

Signs and symptoms of Hyperglycemia

- High blood glucose
- High levels of glucose in the urine
- Frequent urination
- Increased thirst

Causes of Hyperglycemia

- If you have type 1 diabetes, you may not have given yourself enough insulin.
- If you have type 2 diabetes, your body may have enough insulin, but it is not as effective as it should be.
- You ate more than planned or exercised less than planned.
- You have stress from an illness, such as a cold or flu.
- You have other stress, such as family conflicts or school or dating problems.

The effects of hyperglycemia

If you don't treat hyperglycemia, it can become a serious problem, so it's critical to do so as soon as you notice it. Ketoacidosis, often known as a diabetic coma, could develop if hyperglycemia is not treated. When your body doesn't have enough insulin, ketoacidosis develops. Your body breaks down fats to utilize as fuel because it can't utilize glucose without insulin.

Ketones are waste products created when your body breaks down fats. Your body will attempt to eliminate excess ketones through urine because it cannot handle them. Unfortunately, because the body is unable to eliminate all the ketones, they accumulate in your blood and can cause ketoacidosis.

Hyperlipidaemia (high levels of fat in the blood)

Cholesterol is a waxy material, it isn't necessarily "bad" as it is needed by your body to produce hormones, vitamins, and new cells but having too much cholesterol can be harmful. There are two sources of cholesterol, one that can be produced by your liver and the other which is obtained from animal-based diets. For instance, dairy products, pork, and poultry all include dietary cholesterol. They contain a lot of saturated and trans fats. The liver produces more cholesterol than it normally would because of these fats which result in changes in the cholesterol level from healthy to unhealthy because of the increased production. The blood carries cholesterol around in it. The risk to your health increases as your blood's level of cholesterol increases as well which increases the risk of cardiovascular disorders, such as heart disease and stroke, which are associated with high cholesterol.

When it comes to cholesterol, it's crucial to know your numbers. Hyperlipidaemia means your blood has too many lipids (or fats), such as cholesterol and triglycerides. One type of hyperlipidemia, hypercholesterolemia, implies you have too much non-HDL cholesterol and LDL (bad) cholesterol in your blood. This condition increases fatty deposits in arteries and the risk of blockages. Two different lipoproteins transport cholesterol in the body. Low-density lipoprotein, or LDL, is one. High-density lipoprotein, or HDL, is the other. The quantity of each type of cholesterol in your blood is determined by a test.

Low-density Lipoprotein "Bad cholesterol" LDL

Due to its role in the development of fatty deposits in arteries, LDL cholesterol is referred to as the "bad" cholesterol. As a result, the risk of heart attack, stroke, and peripheral arterial disease is increased by the narrowing of the arteries.

High-density lipoprotein "Good cholesterol" HDL

A healthy amount of HDL cholesterol may prevent heart attack and stroke, it is sometimes referred to as "good" cholesterol. LDL (bad) cholesterol is transported by HDL from the arteries back to the liver, where it is digested and eliminated from the body. However, LDL cholesterol is still there even when HDL cholesterol is present. HDL can only carry between one-third and one-fourth of blood cholesterol.

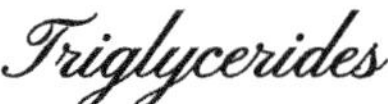

The most prevalent kind of fat in the body is triglyceride. They retain extra calories from your diet. Fat deposits within the artery walls are associated with high triglyceride levels, high LDL (bad) cholesterol, and low HDL (good) cholesterol, which raises the risk of heart attack and stroke.

Another way your cholesterol numbers can be out of balance is when your HDL (good) cholesterol level is too low. With less HDL to eliminate cholesterol from your arteries, your risk of atherosclerotic plaque and blockages increases. The good news is that lowering high cholesterol decreases your chance of developing heart disease and stroke. Have your cholesterol checked if you are 20 years of age or older, and then work with your doctor to change your cholesterol levels as necessary.

Symptoms of diabetes

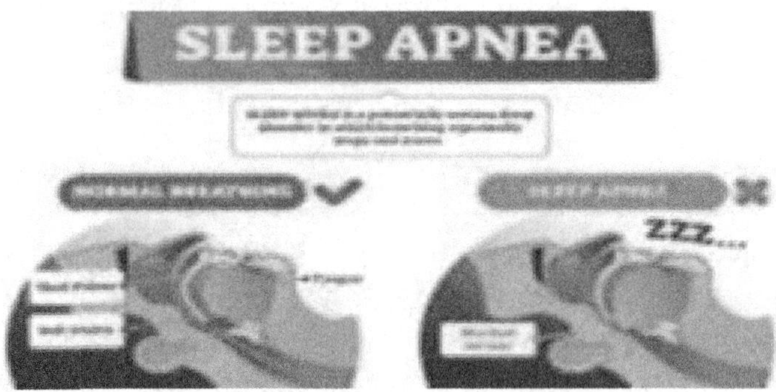

The general symptoms of diabetes include:

- Nausea
- Excessive urination
- Intense hunger
- Intense thirst
- Numbness of limbs
- Reduced resistance to infections
- Blurred
- Weight loss
- Frequent urination
- Extreme fatigue
- ▪ Sores that don't heal

Specific symptoms in men

In addition to the general symptoms of diabetes, men with diabetes may have a decreased sex drive, erectile dysfunction (E.D.), and poor muscle strength due to high blood sugar level that has not been adequately controlled.

Specific symptoms in Women

Women with diabetes can also have symptoms such as urinary tract infections, yeast infections, dry, itchy skin, and an odorous vagina. Sometimes a vaginal infection may be accompanied by vaginal discharges, which are different from normal vaginal discharge.

Unique symptoms of type1 diabetes can include

- Extreme hunger
- Increased thirst
- Deistic weight loss
- Frequent urination
- Blurry vision
- Tiredness

- Occasional mood changes

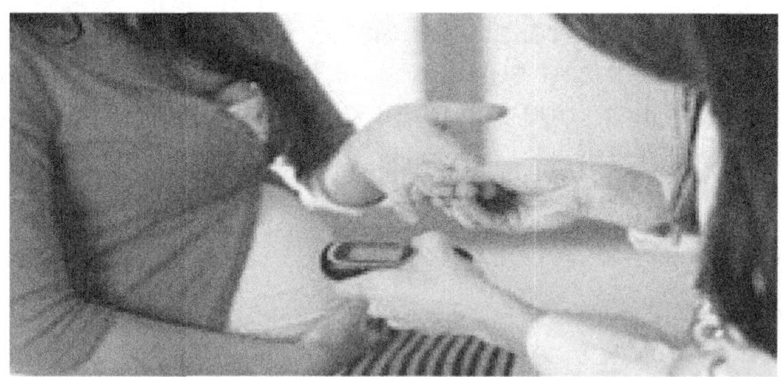

Many women with gestational diabetes don't have any symptoms. The condition is usually detected during a routine blood sugar test or oral glucose tolerance test that is usually performed between the 24th and 28th weeks of gestation or the period of pregnancy.

Sometimes, a woman with gestational diabetes will also experience increased thirst or urination.

The Bottom Line

Diabetes symptoms can be so mild that they are challenging to detect at first. Please, visit your physician if you detect one or two of the symptoms mentioned above.

CHAPTER 2

Prevalence of cardiovascular diseases

Cardiovascular diseases (CVDs) are the leading cause of death globally. According to WHO, 17.9 million deaths worldwide in 2019 were attributable to CVDs, or 32% of all fatalities. Heart attack and stroke deaths accounted for 85% of these fatalities and most CVD fatalities occur in low- and middle-income nations. In 2019, non-communicable illnesses caused 17 million premature deaths (before the age of 70), and 38% of those fatalities were attributable to CVDs.

Addressing behavioral risk factors such as tobacco use, unhealthy eating and obesity, inactivity and problematic alcohol consumption can reduce your risk of developing any of the CVDs however early detection of cardiovascular disease is crucial to start treatment with counseling and medication(cardiovascular diseases (CVDs), n.d.).

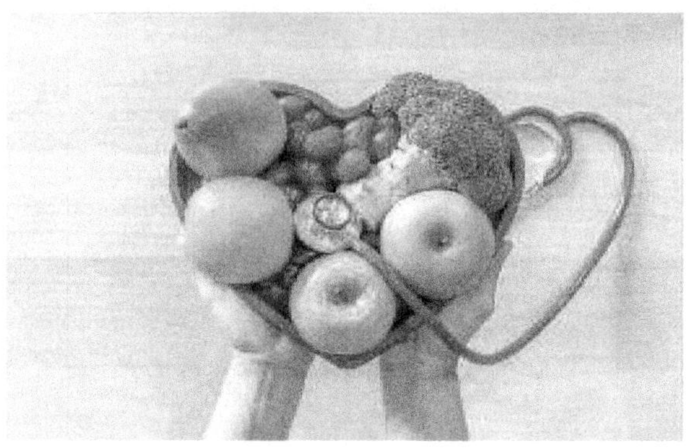

What are cardiovascular diseases

The term "cardiovascular diseases" (CVDs) refers to a variety of heart and blood vessel conditions. They include **Coronary heart disease**, which affects the blood vessels that supply the heart muscle. **Cerebrovascular disease**, which affects the blood vessels that supply the brain, peripheral arterial disease, which affects the blood vessels that supply the arms and legs, **Rheumatic heart disease**, which results from the streptococcal bacteria that cause rheumatic fever-induced inflammation, and scarring damage to the heart muscle and heart valves, which results in rheumatic heart disease. Rheumatic fever is brought on by the body's aberrant response to a streptococcal infection, which typically manifests in children as tonsillitis or sore throats. Children in poor nations, particularly those where poverty is pervasive, are primarily affected by rheumatic fever. Rheumatic heart disease contributes to roughly 2% of cardiovascular disease-related fatalities worldwide.

Shortness of breath, exhaustion, irregular heartbeats, chest pain, and fainting are all signs of rheumatic heart disease.

Rheumatic fever symptoms include fever, joint pain and swelling, nausea, stomach cramps, and vomiting.

Congenital heart disease affects the normal growth and function of the heart from birth.

Deep vein thrombosis and pulmonary embolism such as blood clots in the leg veins can dislodge and move to the heart and lungs. Heart attacks and strokes are typically sudden, severe events that are mostly brought on by a blockage that stops the flow of blood to the heart or brain as a result Fat deposits that have accumulated on the inner walls of the blood arteries that supply the heart or brain also blood clots or hemorrhage from a brain blood artery can result in strokes.

Risk factors of cardiovascular disease

Unhealthy eating, inactivity, usage of tobacco products, and abusing alcohol are the main behavioral risk factors for heart disease and stroke. Individuals may experience elevated blood pressure, elevated blood glucose, and elevated blood lipids, as well as overweight and obesity because of behavioral risk factors. These "intermediate risk variables" can be assessed in primary care settings and point to an elevated risk of consequences like heart attack, stroke, and heart failure. Other additional underlying factors contribute to CVDs. These reflect the three main causes — urbanization, population aging, and globalization — that are causing a social, economic, and cultural transformation. Poverty, stress, and inherited factors are other CVD risk factors.

Additionally, pharmacological therapy for diabetes, high blood lipids, and hypertension is required to lower cardiovascular risk and stop heart attacks and strokes in those who have these disorders.

Symptoms of cardiovascular diseases

- Numbness of the face, arm, or leg, especially on one side of the body.
- Confusion, difficulty speaking or understanding speech. ▪ Difficulty seeing with one or both eyes.

- Difficulty walking, dizziness, and/or loss of balance or coordination.
- Severe headache with no known cause
- Fainting or unconsciousness

CHAPTER 3

When your blood glucose, commonly known as blood sugar, is too high, you develop diabetes. Your primary energy source is blood glucose, which is obtained from the food you eat. The pancreas produces the hormone insulin, which facilitates the entry of food-derived glucose into your cells for energy production. Your body occasionally produces insufficient or no insulin, or it uses insulin poorly. After that, glucose remains in your circulation and does not enter your cells. Over time, health issues might result from having too much glucose in the blood.

Even though there is no treatment for diabetes, you can manage it and maintain your healthIn the United States, 30.3 million people, or 9.4% of the population, had diabetes as of 2015. More than one in four of them were unaware they had the illness. One in four adults over 65 has diabetes. Type 2 diabetes accounts for 90–95 percent of occurrences in adulthood according to the CDC.

Diabetes is occasionally referred to as "borderline diabetes" or "a touch of sugar." These words imply that someone isn't suffering from diabetes.

Types of Diabetes

There are three main types of diabetes

Type 1

Those who have type 1 diabetes cannot produce insulin in their bodies. Your immune system targets and kills the insulin-producing cells in your pancreas. Although it can develop at any age, type 1 diabetes is typically diagnosed in children and young people. To stay alive, people with type 1 diabetes must take insulin every day

Type 2

If you have type 2 diabetes, you may have poor insulin production or usage. Type 2 diabetes can strike at any age, even in infancy. However, those in their middle years and older are most likely to develop this kind of diabetes. These stand as the most prevalent kind of diabetes.

The Dramatic Increase in Type 2 Diabetes

A Tragic Phenomenon Type 2 diabetes occurs in approximately 3 to 5 percent of Americans under fifty years of age and increases to 10 to 15 percent in people over fifty. More than 90 percent of diabetics in the United States are type 2 diabetics. Sometimes called adult-onset diabetes, this form of diabetes occurs most often in people who are overweight and who do not exercise sufficiently. The explosion in the occurrence of diabetes in the last twenty-five years in America parallels the skyrocketing number of overweight people. Type 2 diabetes rarely occurs in people who eat healthily, exercise regularly, and have a low body fat percentage. The disease hardly existed in prior centuries when food was not abundant or when high-calorie, low-nutrient food was not available. It is also more common in people of Native American, Hispanic, Indian, and African American descent, though no background is immune to the effects of a diabetes-inducing diet. Worldwide, diabetes is exploding as populations in all corners of the globe are being exposed to processed foods for the first time in human history. The development and abundance of processed foods in the world's food supply combined with more sedentary jobs have created an explosion of obesity, diabetes, and heart disease. Most countries have attempted to solve this problem with medications for diabetes, high blood pressure, and high cholesterol. Invasive medical procedures and surgeries are used at a substantial expense but without significant lifespan enhancements or benefits to society. In the United States, being overweight is the norm, and almost all adults eventually take prescribed medications for their heart, diabetes, cholesterol, or blood pressure. 51 percent of those over the age of 65 take five or more prescription drugs a day! The number of obese Americans is higher than the number of those who smoke, use illegal drugs, or suffer from other physical ailments. Obesity is a major risk factor associated with highly prevalent serious diseases such as heart disease, cancer, and diabetes. It is what we eat that creates these diseases and fuels out-of-control medical costs. Even five extra pounds on a normal body frame can lead to diabetes. Research shows that excess body fat is the most significant cause of type 2 diabetes. Through working with thousands of patients, I have observed with consistency that losing body fat in conjunction with maintaining high levels of micronutrients in the body's tissues will reduce the need for medications and, in most cases, reverse type 2 diabetes for good. As we'll explore in detail throughout this book, scientific studies show it is not just the weight loss but also the cell's exposure to a favorable micronutrient environment that enables recovery. Many of my patients recover. Many of my patients recover from their diabetes before most of their weight has been lost. The cells become more responsive to insulin when the body is not burdened with excess fat, and the high level of micronutrients in the tissues enables the beta cells that have pooped out from struggling to produce extra high levels of insulin for years to reclaim lost function. Because of its slow onset and the fact that it can usually be controlled with diet, type 2 is considered a milder form of diabetes, sometimes developing over several years. The consequences of uncontrolled and untreated type 2 diabetes, however, are just as serious as those for type 1. Heart attacks, infections, amputations, blindness, and strokes are possible, but unlike type 1, type 2 diabetics can almost all come off insulin and other medications if they take off the excess weight.

Gestational diabetes

This type of diabetes is developed by women during pregnancy. After the baby is born, this type of diabetes typically disappears. However, if you had gestational diabetes, your risk of getting type 2 diabetes in the future is higher. Type 2 diabetes can occasionally be detected during pregnancy.

Gestational diabetes is restricted only to pregnant women. Most pregnant women with gestational diabetes do not show any unique symptoms. It is only diagnosed during a routine blood sugar test or oral glucose tolerance test that is usually performed between the 24th and 28th weeks of gestation. In rare cases, women with gestational Diabetes mellitus only experience increased thirst and urination. Constant urination may be attributed to other conditions, such as resting the enlarged uterus on the pregnant woman's bladder.

Usually, the symptoms of diabetes can be so mild to the extent that they become difficult to be noticed initially. As a result, it is advisable to visit a physician regularly for a checkup, engage in regular physical exercise within the limits of a pregnant woman, and eat enough fruits and vegetables while avoiding junk food.

Different causes are associated with all types of diabetes. It is not yet well known what causes type 1 diabetes. However, for an unknown reason, the immune system may mistakenly attack and destroy insulin-producing beta cells found in the pancreas.

In some people, the gene may play a role in this metabolic process. A virus may also be responsible for setting off the immune system attack.

Symptoms of Gestational Diabetes

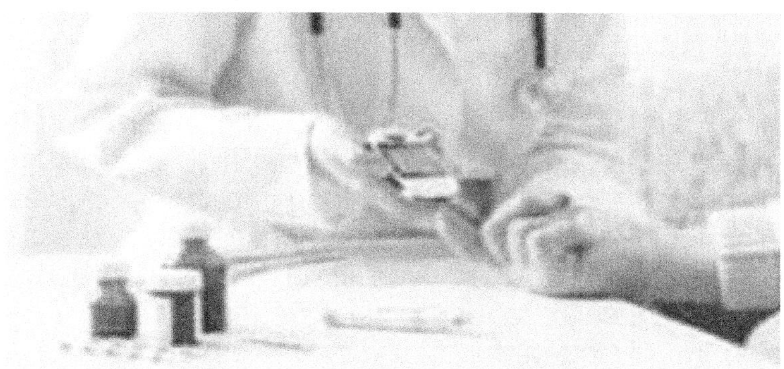

There are many general symptoms of gestational diabetes. These include

- Increased thirst
- Intense hunger
- Frequent urination
- Progressive weight loss
- Extreme fatigue
- Blurry/poor vision
- Sore that is difficult to heal

In males, where pregnancy does not occur, specific diabetic symptoms are peculiar. These symptoms are not noticed in females. They include:

- Decreased libido is where the urge for sexual intercourse wanes in the man.
- Erectile dysfunction is when the man cannot achieve a penile erection or a weak erection that will be unable to achieve vaginal penetration. Sometimes, when erection is

achieved, it is not sustained for any meaningful coition or sexual intercourse.

- Poor muscle strength

All these symptoms are attributed to the inelastic nature and narrowing of the blood vessels due to the high blood sugar level. These obstruct the smooth flow of blood into the spongy tissues of the penis, inhibiting penile erection, unsustained erection, and reduced libido in males. In type 2 diabetes, the body cannot effectively use insulin to bring glucose to the cells through its conversion to glycogen for storage. Consequently, the body is compelled to look for an alternative energy source.

Diabetic neuropathy is also called diabetic peripheral neuropathy. The cause is a long-term high blood sugar level that later causes nerve damage. Some will not show any symptoms, but in some patients, the symptoms may be debilitating. According to the USA National Institute for Diabetes, 60% to 70% of patients with digestive tract and kidney disease have some form of neuropathy.

The most common form of diabetic neuropathy is peripheral neuropathy which affects body extremities such as legs, feet, toes, and arms. The major problem in the control and care of diabetes is that many people do not know that they have diabetes. When people are unaware of their diabetes status, they cannot associate the unusual sensation they experience in the various parts of their bodies with diabetes. Most forms of erectile dysfunction are caused by diabetic neuropathy. Unfortunately, many patients do not care to know the primary cause of their sexual impotence but resort to aphrodisiacs until the onset of complications. Men who have erectile dysfunction should, first of all, establish their diabetes status before taking aphrodisiacs which may provide temporary relief to their problem.

What causes diabetic nerve damage

High blood sugar level that has existed for an extended period is the leading cause of damage to nerve endings. Why and how high blood sugar levels cause nerve damage is not yet known. One possible reason is the intricate interplay between the blood vessels and nerves, according to NIDDK.

Other factors perceived to be responsible include high blood pressure, high cholesterol levels, and nerve inflammation. Diabetic peripheral neuropathy appears first in the feet and legs and later in the arms.

Feeling numbness

Numbness is a common symptom of diabetic peripheral neuropathy. A diabetic patient suffering from peripheral neuropathy may sometimes be unable to feel that they are walking while walking. There may also be a tingling and burning sensation in the hands and feet or a feeling of wearing a sock while no socks are worn on any of the feet. That is why such an individual may be cut on the feet or arm without feeling it. Such injury also makes it difficult to heal and may lead to amputation of such a limb. Patients should always wear protective footwear and be careful not to sustain avoidable physical injuries.

Where is diabetes more prevalent

Four out of five people in the world with diabetes now live in low- and middle-income countries (LMIC), and the incidence of diabetes is increasing in poorer communities. Diabetes increases susceptibility to infection and worsens outcomes for some of the world's major infectious diseases, such as tuberculosis, melioidosis, and dengue. However, the relationship between diabetes and many neglected tropical diseases is yet to be adequately quantified. There is some evidence that chronic viral infections such as hepatitis B and HIV may predispose an individual to the development of type 2 diabetes by chronic inflammatory and immune metabolic mechanisms. Helminth infections such as schistosomiasis may be protective against the development of diabetes. This finding opens up new territory for discovering novel therapeutics for the prevention and treatment of diabetes.

A greater understanding of the impact of diabetes on risks and outcomes for infections causing significant diseases in LMIC is necessary to develop vaccines and therapies for the increasing number of people with diabetes at risk of infection and to pay more attention to research works as well as public health interventions and policy. I have been able to explain the current international diabetes prevalence, the evidence for interactions between diabetes and infection, immune mechanisms for the interaction, and potential interventions to combat the co-infection of diabetes and other on-diabetic infections such as dengue, melioidosis, tropical and tuberculosis.

About 336 million people with diabetes are now living in low and middle-income countries (LMIC). Types 1 and 2 diabetes increase susceptibility to infection and worsen the outcomes for diseases such as tuberculosis (T.B.). Current international treatment guidelines for diabetes are based on research conducted in high-income countries focused on preventing adverse cardiovascular diseases and early death. There is no empirical evidence to base guidelines for people living in LMIC, where there is an increased incidence of infectious diseases compared with high-income countries.

Pregnancy (Gestational) diabetes

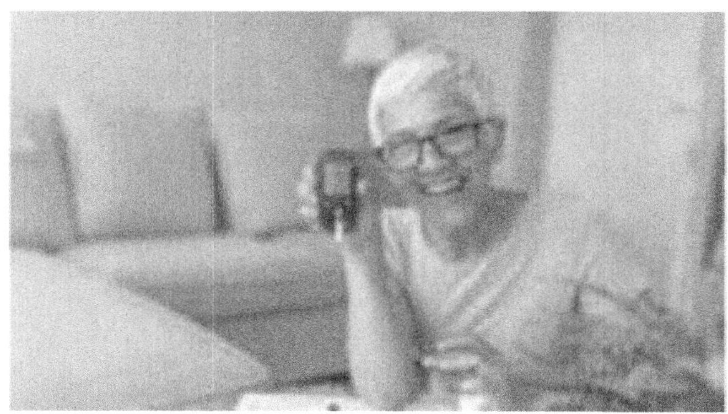

Diabetes mellitus, which occurs during pregnancy, is called gestational diabetes. That is usually temporary and disappears as soon as the woman gives birth. It can be managed until the woman delivers her baby. The pregnant woman should be active during and after pregnancy.

Children (Neonatal) Diabetes

Diabetes Mellitus in children is referred to as neonatal diabetes. Most neonatal diabetes cases are type 1 diabetes. Some are due to infant obesity caused by overnutrition. That accounts for the high rate of infant diabetes in children born to the most affluent homes, especially in Africa and Asia.

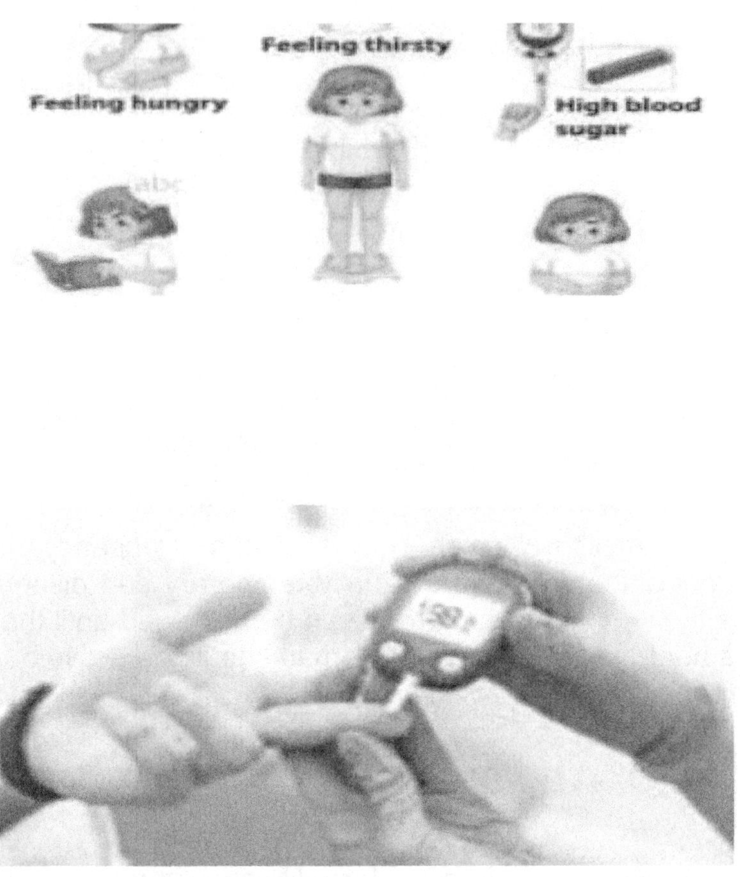

Pre-diabetes

It occurs when your blood sugar is slightly higher than usual but is not high enough for a diagnosis of type 2 diabetes.

A rare condition called diabetes insipidus is not related to Diabetes mellitus, although it has a similar name. It is a different condition in which the kidneys remove too much fluid from the body. Each type of diabetes has unique symptoms, causes, and treatments.

Monogenic forms of diabetes

Some uncommon types of diabetes, known as monogenic diabetes, are caused by mutations or alterations in a single gene. Monogenic types of diabetes make up 1 to 4% of all cases of diabetes in the United States. The gene mutation that causes monogenic diabetes is typically inherited from one or both parents. Sometimes the gene mutation appears on its own; in this case, neither parent carries the mutation. Most mutations that result in monogenic diabetes decrease the body's capacity to make insulin, a pancreatic protein that aids in the body's utilization of glucose as fuel. Most cases of monogenic diabetes are misdiagnosed. For instance, type 2 diabetes is frequently identified rather than monogenic diabetes when elevated blood glucose levels are first noticed in adults. Genetic testing may be required to diagnose and determine the kind of monogenic diabetes if your doctor suspects you may have it. To find out if other family members are at risk for or already have a monogenic form of diabetes that is passed down from generation to generation, testing may be necessary. While certain types of monogenic diabetes can be managed with oral diabetes medications (pills), others call for insulin injections. A thorough diagnosis enables effective therapy, which can eventually result in better glucose regulation and long-term health. There are two main types of monogenic diabetes which include.

Neonatal diabetes mellitus (NDM)

This monogenic form of diabetes called NDM appears in infants between the ages of 6 and 12 months. Up to 1 in 400,000 infants in the US have NDM, making it a rare illness. Infants with NDM do not produce enough insulin, which causes their blood sugar levels to rise. NDM is sometimes confused for type 1 diabetes, while type 1 diabetes seldom manifests before the age of six months. Nearly always, diabetes that develops in the first six months of infancy is hereditary in origin. Numerous genes and mutations that can cause NDM had been found by researchers. About 50% of NDM patients have a permanent condition known as permanent neonatal diabetes mellitus. The disease, known as persistent neonatal diabetes mellitus, is lifelong in around half of those with NDM. The remaining cases of NDM are characterized by a transitory, or brief, a disease that usually goes away during infancy but may later resurface.

Symptoms of NDM

The individual's gene mutations determine the clinical characteristics of NDM.

- Frequent urination, fast breathing, and dehydration are symptoms of NDM.
- Elevated blood or urine glucose levels can be used to diagnose 5 NDM.

A potentially fatal disease known as diabetic ketoacidosis may develop from the body producing molecules called ketones due to a lack of insulin.

Intrauterine growth restriction is the medical term for the fact that most babies with NDM do not develop normally in pregnancy and that newborns with NDM are substantially smaller than those of the same gestational age. After birth, some babies don't acquire weight or develop as quickly as babies of their age and sex.

The right kind of Management could enhance and normalize growth and development.

Maturity onset diabetes of the Young (MODY)

A monogenic form of diabetes called MODY typically develops throughout adolescence or the early stages of adulthood. Up to 2% of all diabetes cases in people 20 years of age and under in the US are caused by MODY. It has been linked to a variety of gene mutations, all of which reduce the pancreas' capacity to generate insulin. High blood glucose levels result from this, which over time may harm bodily tissues, especially the kidneys, eyes, nerves, and blood vessels. Either type 1 or type 2 may be confused with MODY. In the past, persons with MODY typically did not have obesity, overweight, or other type 2 diabetes risks factors such as high blood pressure or unusual blood fat levels. However, people with MODY may also be overweight or obese as the number of obese or overweight Americans rises.

Although both type 2 diabetes and MODY can run in families, those who have it often have a history of the disease in several generations, which means they have it in their grandparents, parents, and children.

The individual's gene mutations determine the clinical characteristics of MODY.

People who carry specific mutations may have mildly elevated blood sugar levels that remain steady throughout their lives, minimal or no signs of diabetes, and no long-term consequences. Only standard blood testing may reveal their elevated blood glucose levels. Other mutations, however, demand specialized care, either with insulin or a class of oral diabetic drugs known as sulfonylureas.

How to diagnose NDM & MODY

Most types of monogenic diabetes can be diagnosed by genetic testing.

Genetic testing is advised if diabetes is discovered within the first six months of life.

Long-term glycaemic control and health improvements should result from a precise diagnosis and appropriate therapy.

Diabetes is diagnosed in children and young adults, especially those with a strong family history of the disease, who do not have the typical symptoms of type 1 or type 2 diabetes, such as the presence of diabetes-related autoantibodies, obesity, and other metabolic features. Instead, they have stable, mild fasting hyperglycemia, especially if obesity is absent.

A blood or saliva sample must be provided for genetic testing for monogenic diabetes so that DNA can be isolated. For mutations in the genes that lead to monogenic diabetes, the DNA is examined. Specialist labs conduct genetic testing.

A person's gene for diabetes can be identified by abnormal results, as can the likelihood that they would eventually acquire a monogenic form of diabetes. The best suitable course of treatment for those with monogenic diabetes can be determined with the use of genetic testing. Testing is crucial while preparing for pregnancy and understanding the possibility of passing on monogenic diabetes to a future child if you, your spouse, or other family members have the disease.

Risk factors of Diabetes

If you are overweight, older than 45, or have a family history of diabetes, you are more likely to acquire type 2 diabetes. Your likelihood of getting type 2 diabetes is also influenced by your level of physical inactivity, race, and several medical conditions like high blood pressure. If you have prediabetes or had gestational diabetes while you were pregnant, you are also more likely to acquire type 2 diabetes. Find out more about the dangers of type 2 diabetes.

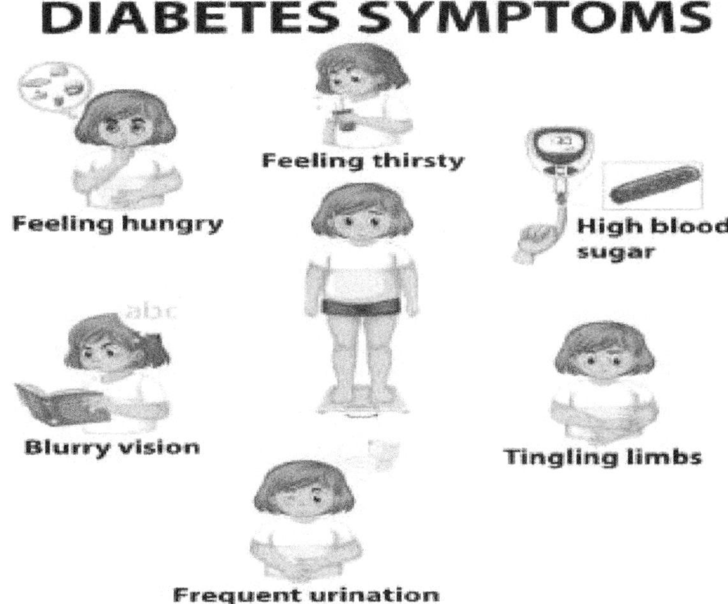

Effect of Diabetes

According to the American Heart Association, those with diabetes have a risk of cardiovascular disease that is more than double that of the general population. Heart disease is the leading cause of death for those with type 2 diabetes. Diabetes patients' excessive blood glucose (sugar) levels over time can harm both the nerves that control their blood vessels and their blood vessels themselves.

Sugar is normally used by body tissues as an energy source. It is kept as a type of glycogen in the liver. Diabetes can cause blood sugar to remain in the bloodstream and leak from the liver into the blood, damaging your blood vessels and the nerves that regulate them. Blood flow and nutrient supply to your heart might be slowed down or stopped by a blocked coronary artery. The longer you have diabetes, the higher your risk of heart disease. Untreated diabetes can affect some of the organs and will result in a lot of complications. One of the most prevalent risk factors for heart disease in diabetics is high blood pressure as it damages your blood vessels and puts your heart under stress. You become more prone to several issues as a result, such as:

- heart attack
- stroke
- kidney problems
- vision issues

Heart attack

If the vessels in your body are damaged by diabetes, you could experience a heart attack if a portion of your heart muscle isn't getting enough blood.

People with diabetes are more likely than those without diabetes to develop heart failure after having a heart attack. Heart failure, which results from the heart's inability to pump enough blood to the body, is more likely to develop in diabetics. One of the most dangerous cardiovascular consequences of diabetes is heart failure.

The following are possible heart attack symptoms:

- Pain in the chest, weakness, or dizziness

- Particularly in women having a heart attack, you may experience nausea, vomiting, and extraordinary exhaustion as well as pain or discomfort in your arms, shoulders, back, neck, or jaw.
- Breathing difficulty
- ▪ Swelling in the legs, feet, and ankles coughing and fatigue

Stroke

When a blood vessel in the brain is blocked or breaks, a stroke happens. Adults with diabetes are 1.5 times more likely to experience a stroke than those without the disease because a stroke disrupts the flow of blood and oxygen to the brain, which can harm brain tissue. Your body's ability to effectively metabolize food is hampered by diabetes. Because of a lack of insulin production or improper insulin usage, your blood glucose (sugar) levels increase. The blood arteries in the body can become damaged over time by high glucose levels, which raises the risk of stroke.

Symptoms of stroke

- Difficulty speaking or understanding speech.
- Memory loss.
- Numbness or paralysis (inability to move).
- Pain.
- Problems controlling or expressing emotions, or depression.
- Trouble thinking, paying attention, learning, or making judgments.
- Sometimes death.

Kidney problems

Blood arteries in your kidneys can become damaged by high blood glucose, often known as blood sugar. Blood vessels are less effective when they are damaged. High blood pressure is a common complication of diabetes, and it can harm your kidneys. Kidney damage is more likely to occur if you have diabetes for a longer period. If you have diabetes, kidney disease is more likely to develop if your blood sugar levels are too high or your blood pressure is too high.

Diabetes, renal disease, and kidney failure are more common in African Americans, American Indians, and Hispanics/Latinos than in Caucasians.

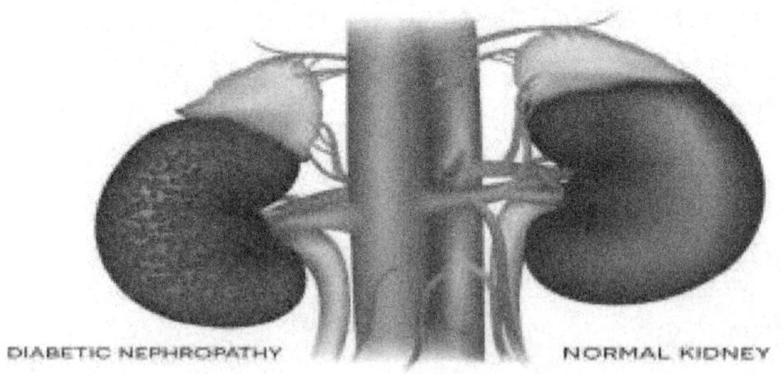

Most diabetic kidney disease sufferers do not exhibit any symptoms. Getting your kidneys examined is the only method to determine if you have diabetic renal disease.

Blood and urine tests are used by medical practitioners to look for diabetic kidney damage. To determine how well your kidneys are filtering your blood, your doctor will check your urine for albumin and perform a blood test.

If you have type 2 diabetes or have had type 1 diabetes for more than five years, you should get tested for kidney disease annually.

Vision problems

Over time, diabetes can harm your eyes, resulting in vision loss or possibly blindness. The good news is that diabetes management and routine eye exams can help prevent visual issues and halt their progression.

Diabetes patients are susceptible to developing diabetic retinopathy, macular edema (which typically occurs in conjunction with diabetic retinopathy), cataracts, and glaucoma. All these conditions can cause vision loss, but early detection and treatment can greatly improve your chances of keeping your sight.

Retina nephropathy

High blood sugar destroys the retina's blood vessels, which results in diabetic retinopathy. Blood flow may be halted, or eyesight may become fuzzy because of swollen, leaking, damaged blood vessels. New blood vessels can occasionally form, but they aren't always healthy and can worsen existing visual issues. Both eyes are typically affected by diabetic retinopathy. There are two stages of retina nephropathy in diabetic patients.

Diabetic Retinopathy

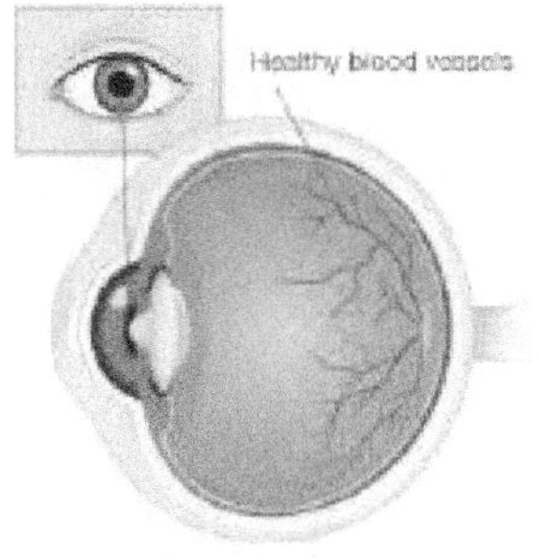

Normal Eye

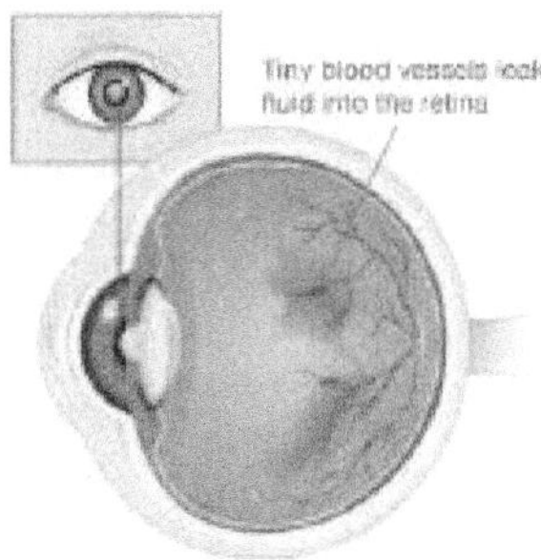

Eye with Retinopathy

Early stage (non-proliferative): Retinal blood vessel walls sag and enlarge, generating minute pouches (you won't be able to see them, but an ophthalmologist can). These pouches have the potential to leak blood and other fluids, which could cause the macula, a region of the retina, to expand (macular edema), blurring your vision. The most frequent reason for blindness in those with diabetic retinopathy is macular edema. Macular edema develops in about half of the diabetic retinopathy patients.

Proliferative stage: At this stage, the retina starts to sprout new blood vessels. Because they are weak, these young arteries frequently bleed into the vitreous. You might notice a few floating, dark dots in your eyesight if there is mild bleeding. The amount of bleeding could completely obstruct your vision.

Symptoms in the advanced stage can include:

- Blurry vision
- Spots or dark shapes in your vision (floaters)
- Trouble seeing colors
- Dark or empty areas in your vision
- Vision loss

CHAPTER 4

Cancer

Cancer is a condition when a few of the body's cells grow out of control and spread to other bodily regions. In the millions of cells that make up the human body, cancer can develop practically anywhere. Human cells often divide (via a process known as cell growth and multiplication) to create new cells as the body requires them. New cells replace old ones when they die because of aging or damage. Occasionally, this systematic process fails, causing damaged or aberrant cells to proliferate when they shouldn't. Tumors, which are tissue masses, can develop from these cells. Tumors may or may not be malignant(What Is Cancer? - NCI, n.d.)

Development of cancer

Cancer is a genetic disease—that is, it is caused by alterations to genes that control the way our cells behave, notably how they grow and divide.

- Errors that occur during cell division can lead to genetic alterations that cause cancer.

- DNA deterioration brought on by unfavorable environmental elements including the toxins in tobacco smoke and the sun's UV radiation.
- They were inherited to the US by our parents.

Types of cancers

Proto-oncogenes, tumor suppressor genes, and DNA repair genes are the three primary gene groups that are typically impacted by the genetic alterations that cause cancer. These modifications are commonly referred to as cancer's "drivers."

Proto-oncogenes play a role in regular cell division and proliferation. However, these genes may develop into cancer-causing genes (or oncogenes), allowing cells to grow and survive when they shouldn't by being changed in specific ways or being more active than usual.

Genes that decrease tumors are also involved in regulating cell division and proliferation. Certain tumor suppressor gene mutations can cause cells to divide uncontrollably.

DNA damage must be repaired using DNA repair genes. It is common for cells with mutations in these genes to also have mutations in other genes and chromosomal abnormalities including duplications and deletions of chromosomal segments.

These alterations might work together to turn the cells malignant.

There are over 100 different cancers exist. Typically, cancer types are called for the organs or tissues in which they first appear. For instance, brain cancer begins in the brain, and lung cancer begins in the lung. The type of cell that gave rise to cancer, such as an epithelial cell or a squamous cell, can also be used to describe the condition.

Cancers and diabetes

In addition to having a higher risk of heart disease or renal disease, people with diabetes, especially Type 2 diabetes, also have a higher risk of developing cancer.

- Breast cancer
- Endometrial cancer
- Colorectal cancer
- Liver Cancer

Prostate cancer risk is decreased in people with type 2 diabetes. This could be because some diabetic men have lower levels of the male hormone testosterone in their bodies while people with type 1 diabetes are at a higher risk of developing cervix and stomach cancer however researchers are unsure if this is due to the various health issues that frequently accompany diabetes, like obesity, or the way that aberrant insulin levels increase your risk of developing cancer. Obesity, inflammation, and elevated blood sugar are all linked to diabetes and cancer. If you have diabetes, controlling your blood sugar levels is the best thing you can do.

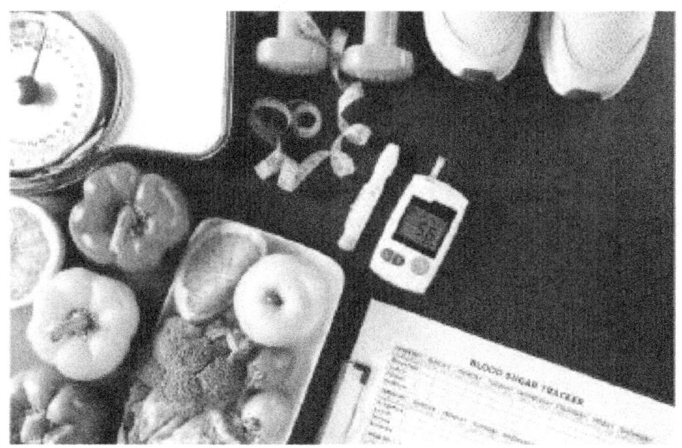

CHAPTER 5

Ways to Manage Diabetes

If you have been diagnosed with diabetes already, advice for managing or reducing your risk of acquiring type 2 diabetes is equally relevant. All these non-communicable diseases are lifestyle diseases therefore some factors can be controlled and so to avoide these conditions are as follows:

Control your weight or maintain a healthy weight

The most significant contributing factor to type 2 diabetes is being overweight. Type 2 diabetes is seven times more likely to develop if you are overweight. Diabetes is 20–40 times more likely to occur in obese people than in healthy-weight people.

If your weight is above the healthy weight range, losing weight may assist. Your odds of acquiring type 2 diabetes can be reduced in half by losing 7– 10% of your present weight and this can be done by Getting up and leaving the television alone.

Type 2 diabetes is promoted by inactivity

Your muscles' capacity to utilize insulin and absorb glucose is improved by working them more frequently and making them work harder. Your insulin-producing cells are less under stress as a result. So, switch up some of your sitting time for exercise. For this benefit, it is not required to engage in protracted hot, sweating exercises.

According to data from the Nurses' Health Study and the Health Professionals Follow-up Study, vigorous daily walking for 30 minutes lowers the incidence of type 2 diabetes by 30%. More recently, The Black Women's Health Study revealed comparable benefits of brisk walking for more than 5 hours per week in terms of avoiding diabetes. Other advantages of this level of activity are numerous. Additionally, more frequent, and intensive exercise can result in even greater cardiovascular and other benefits.

Watching television seems to be a particularly harmful form of inactivity: For every two hours you spend doing so instead of doing anything more active, your risk of acquiring diabetes rises by 20%, along with your risk of heart disease (15%) and early mortality (13%). People who watch more television are more likely to be overweight or obese, which appears to partially account for the relationship between TV watching and diabetes. The bad eating habits linked to TV viewing such as the consumption of unhealthy of snacks may also contribute to the explanation of this relationship (Tanasescu et al., 2003).

Healthy eating

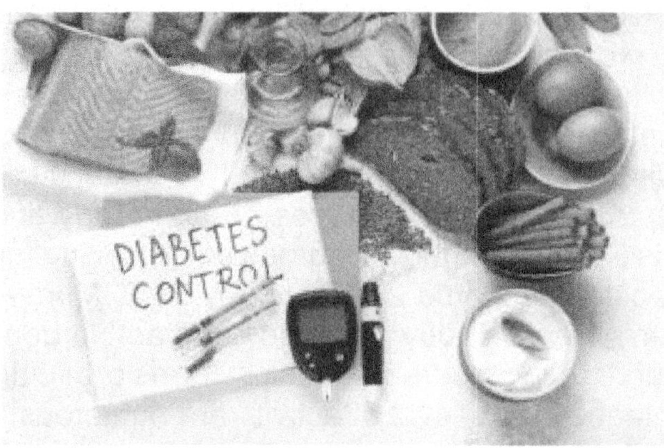

Good nutrition is a primary aspect of healthy living but eating healthy meals and avoiding junk foods can be quite challenging There is no special nutrient found in whole grains that prevents diabetes and enhances health. Everything must be in place and function as a whole; this is crucial. Whole grains' bran and fiber make it more challenging for digestive enzymes to convert starches into glucose. A lower glycaemic index and lower, slower spikes in blood sugar and insulin are the results of this. They lessen the burden on the body's insulin-producing system as a result, which may aid in the prevention of type 2 diabetes. [9] Additionally, whole grains are a good source of phytochemicals, vital vitamins, and minerals that may help lower the risk of diabetes. There is strong evidence that whole grain diets reduce the chance of developing diabetes, but diets high in refined carbs raise the risk (de Munter et al., 2007; Rank et al., 2001). For instance, in the Nurses' Health Studies I and II, researchers examined the consumption of whole grains among more than 160,000 women whose health and eating patterns were monitored for up to 18 years. Compared to women who rarely ate whole grains, those who consumed an average of 2-3 servings of whole grains per day had a 30% lower risk of type 2 diabetes(Alessa et al., 2015). The researchers discovered that consuming an additional two servings of whole grains per day reduced the incidence of type 2 diabetes by 21% when they merged these findings with those of six other sizable trials. Recent research from the Nurses Health Studies I and II and the Health Professionals Follow-Up Study suggests that switching from white rice to whole grains may help reduce the chance of developing diabetes: The risk of developing diabetes was shown to be 17% greater in both women and men who consumed the whitest rice—five or more servings per week—compared to those who consumed it less frequently. Two or more servings of brown rice per week or more were associated with an 11% decreased risk of developing diabetes than eating little to no brown rice. According to research, substituting whole grains for even a small amount of white rice could reduce the risk of diabetes by 36%(Alessa et al., 2015).

Fresh vegetables – The best choices are fresh, frozen, and canned vegetables and vegetable juices without added sodium, fat, or sugar. Try to eat at least 3-5 daily servings of vegetables, including asparagus, broccoli, cabbage, carrots, cauliflower, celery, eggplant, greens, peppers, snap peas, and tomatoes. A serving of vegetables is ½ cup of cooked vegetables or vegetable juice; or 1 cup of raw vegetables.

Fruits – Eat fruits that are fresh, frozen, or canned without added sugars. Common fruits include apples, blackberries, blueberries, cantaloupe, dates, figs, grapes, oranges, pears, and strawberries.

Replace sugary drinks, coffees, and teas with water

Sugary drinks have a high glycemic load, like refined grains, and consuming more of this sweet stuff is linked to a higher risk of developing diabetes. According to the Nurses' Health Study II, type 2 diabetes risk was 83% greater for women who drank one or more sugar-sweetened beverages per day than for those who drank less than one per month similarly other studies also indicate that fruit drinks, including juices, fortified fruit drinks, and powdered drinks, may not be as healthy as they are frequently portrayed to be in food commercials. According to the Black Women's Health study, women who consumed two or more fruit drinks per day had a 31% higher risk of developing type 2 diabetes than those who consumed fewer than one serving per month(de Koning et al., 2011).

How do sugary beverages cause this elevated risk? A relationship could be explained by weight gain. Women who consumed more sugary beverages gained greater weight than those who consumed fewer sugary beverages in both the Nurses' Health Study II and the Black Women's Health Study. According to numerous studies, children and adults who consume soda or other drinks with added sugar are more likely to acquire weight than those who do not, and replacing them with unsweetened beverages or water will help you lose weight however, the increased risk of diabetes may not entirely be attributed to weight gain brought on by sugary beverages(Vartanian et al., 2007). There is growing proof that sugary beverages cause long-term inflammation, high triglycerides, decreased "good" (HDL) cholesterol, and increase risk of diabetes and other non communicable diseases. What can I substitute for sweet beverages? Water is a great option only if you don't overdo it on the sugar and cream, coffee and tea are also excellent calorie-free alternatives to sweetened beverages(Malik et al., 2010).

Choose healthy fats

Diabetes development can also be influenced by the types of fats you consume. Nuts, seeds, and liquid vegetable oils, which include polyunsaturated fats, are examples of healthy fats that can help prevent types 2 diabetes(Mozaffarian et al., 2006). Trans fats have the opposite effect. Most fast-food restaurants' fried dishes, packaged baked goods, numerous types of margarine, and any item with the labeling "partially hydrogenated vegetable oil" included these dangerous fats in the past. Even though there is ample evidence that these marine omega 3 fats help prevent heart disease, eating polyunsaturated fats from fish, sometimes referred to as "long chain omega 3" or "marine omega 3" fats, does not protect against diabetes. Eating fish can help protect you from developing diabetes if you already have it and protect you against other non-communicable diseases(Risérus et al., 2009).

Low-fat or non-fat dairy products – Choose fat-free or low-fat (1%) milk, non-fat yogurt (without added sugar), and unflavoured soy milk.

Lean meats – The best choices are cuts of meats and meat alternatives that are lower in saturated fat and calories. Include fish and seafood, poultry without the skin, eggs, and choice grades of meats trimmed of fat. Most importantly, be sure to watch portion sizes.

Reduce red meat and processed meat consumption

The risk of developing diabetes was reduced by up to 35% by replacing red meat or processed red meat with a better protein source, such as nuts, low-fat dairy, chicken, fish, or whole grains. Unsurprisingly, giving up processed red meat resulted in the largest risk reductions. The evidence that eating red meat (beef, hog, and lamb) and processed red meat (bacon, hot dogs, and deli meats) increase the risk of developing diabetes, even in those who consume just little amounts, is becoming more and more compelling. Researchers have discovered that consuming just one 3- ounce meal of red meat per day—roughly the size of a deck of cards in steak—increased the risk of type 2 diabetes by 20%. eating just two slices of bacon and one hot dog every day increases your risk of diabetes by 51%. Why do various kinds of meat seem to increase the risk of diabetes? It's possible that red meat's high iron content reduces insulin's efficiency or harms the cells that make insulin. It's also possible that processed red meat's high salt and nitrite (a preservative) content is to blame. The unwholesome "Western" eating pattern, which tends to cause diabetes in persons who are already at genetic risk, is characterized by red and processed meats. Additionally, a body of research in a related field has suggested that plant-based eating habits may reduce the risk of type 2 diabetes, and more specifically, that people who follow primarily healthy plant-based diets may have a lower risk of developing type 2 diabetes than people who follow these diets with a lower level of adherence.

Reduce alcohol consumption

For type 2 diabetes, the same might be true. Alcohol use in moderation— up to one drink per day for women and two for men— improves insulin's ability to transport glucose into cells. Additionally, some research shows that moderate alcohol use lowers the risk of type 2 diabetes, although consuming too much alcohol raises the danger. If you already consume alcohol, it's important to keep your intake reasonable because excessive amounts could raise your chance of developing diabetes(Djoussé et al., 2007). You can have the same advantages if you don't consume alcohol by decreasing weight, increasing your level of exercise, and altering your dietary habits. Add type 2 diabetes to the long list of health problems linked with smoking. Smokers are roughly 50% more likely to develop diabetes than non-smokers, and heavy smokers have an even higher risk.

In conclusion, diabetes is a chronic disease that can be effectively controlled for healthy living; adhering to all dietary recommendations and engaging in 15 to 30 minutes of physical activity each day will improve your health and lower your risk of developing diabetic complications. This book gives readers many resources to choose from for additional information on the nutritional treatment of diabetes. Finish this book, and you'll live a long time with properly controlled blood sugar levels without experiencing any problems.

CHAPTER 6

Diabetes mellitus can be controlled if it is not curable. However, recent scientific findings have shown that the disease can be controlled with the appropriate technology with the recent advancement in science and technology, especially in Molecular Biology and Genetic Engineering. Exercise increases the insulin sensitivity of your cells, meaning that you need less insulin to manage your blood sugar level.

Many types of physical activity have been shown to reduce insulin resistance and blood sugar in adults with pre-diabetes or type 2 diabetes. These include aerobic exercise and high-intensity or brisk walking. All these will help to reduce the prevalence of diabetes.

Management of kidney complications from type1 diabetes

Management of kidney complications from Type1 diabetes is done by: Eliminating the need for insulin injections Reducing or eliminating the need for dietary and activity restrictions Reducing or eliminating the risk of severely low blood sugar levels.

Eligibility

A pancreas transplant should not be recommended for patients who can manage their diabetes through diet, medication, and other means since the procedure carries all the risks and recovery issues of major surgery, as well as the possibility that the body's immune system may reject the transplanted organ. To prevent organ rejection, transplant recipients must take powerful immunosuppressant medications for the rest of their lives. The medication has many side effects and makes patients more susceptible to other illnesses.

Patients with Type 1 diabetes may be evaluated for pancreas transplants or combined kidney-pancreas transplants. Patients with Type 2 diabetes are less likely to be candidates because they may be insulin-resistant, meaning that their body's cells do not respond typically to insulin and would not reap the benefits of a pancreas transplant.

Evaluation

When you become insulin dependent, you depend on an external source for insulin injections; usually, at age 18 or older, you will need blood tests to measure your levels of C-peptide. C-peptide is a product of insulin production. There will be several other medical tests as part of your evaluation, such as:

- Blood tests, including an HIV test, were performed last year ▪ Chest X-ray performed within the last year
- Creatinine clearance testing for that not on dialysis. This 24-hour test measures the
- Levels of a blood waste product called creatinine in the blood and urine and is used to evaluate kidney function.
- An echocardiogram was performed within the last two years

- Electrocardiogram performed within the last year

We are presenting thallium or comparable test performed within the last two years.

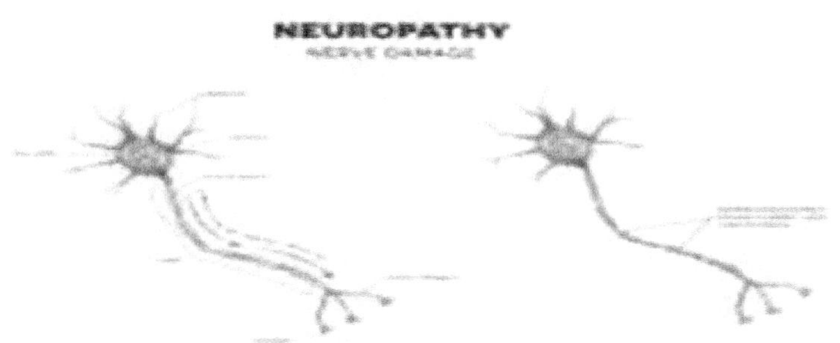

This test involves receiving two substances via IV: Persantine to help expand the arteries and replicate the effect of vigorous exercise, and thallium, a radioactive isotope detected by X-ray (US. FDA, 2021).

Pancreas Transplantation

Pancreas transplantation is a type of surgery in which you receive a healthy donor pancreas. A pancreas transplant is a choice for some people with Type 1 diabetes. Type 1 diabetes is an autoimmune disease in which the pancreas stops producing the hormone insulin. The usual treatment for type 1 diabetes involves daily injections of insulin.

During a pancreas transplant, you will receive a healthy pancreas from a donor who has died. If you have kidney failure from your diabetes, your surgeon may also do a kidney transplant at the same time. The kidney transplant may be done earlier or even after the pancreas transplant. In a pancreas transplant, your pancreas remains in your body. The surgeon generally connects the new pancreas to your intestines so its digestive juices can drain. After a successful transplant, you will no longer need to take insulin. Instead, the new pancreas will create insulin for you. You can eat a regular diet, like an average person. You will have few or no episodes of low or very high blood sugar or insulin shock, and your risk for kidney damage will decrease.

Who is a candidate for the transplant?

Candidates for pancreas transplantation generally have Type 1 diabetes, usually along with kidney damage, nerve damage, eye problems, or other complications. In this case, healthcare providers consider a transplant for someone whose diabetes is out of control, even with medical treatment. That is true, especially when low blood sugar, and hypoglycemia, have persisted for a long time. Some selected people with Type 2 diabetes have received pancreas transplants as well. A pancreas transplant also works best on people without heart or blood vessel disease. If you choose a pancreas transplant, you may be asked to stop smoking or lose weight before the surgery.

What are the risks?

The risks involved in this procedure are infection and organ rejection. Rejection happens when the body's immune system attacks the new organ as a "foreign" invader. To reduce the chances of rejection, the healthcare team tries to match the blood and tissue type of the organ donor to the person getting the transplant, otherwise called the recipient.

After the transplant, healthcare providers prescribe medicines that suppress the immune system, such as azathioprine and cyclosporine, to help prevent the rejection of the new pancreas. However, these medicines make it more likely for people with a transplanted organ to pick up infections like colds and flu. Over time, the medicines may also increase the risk for certain cancers. As a result of the higher risk for skin cancer, for example, it is essential to cover up and wear sunscreen. If you get a pancreas transplant, you must take particular medicines as long as you have the transplanted organ in your body. You will also need tests over the years to be sure that your pancreas transplant is functioning adequately. It is also crucial to keep all your healthcare provider appointments.

Is there a waiting list?

Presently, more people need a healthy pancreas than can be provided for by donors. The wait for a pancreas can be long and averages about 3 years.

Surgeons may plan to do a pancreas transplant at the same time as a kidney transplant to help to control blood glucose levels and reduce damage to the new kidney. The rate of rejection is less if the immune characteristics of the donated organ match more and are capable of existing with those of the patient who receives the transplant or organ recipient.

What is the outlook after a pancreas transplant?

The long-term outlook for persons who receive a pancreas transplant is quite good. Persons who receive simultaneous kidney-pancreas transplants also tend to have less chance of rejection. A positive long-term result depends on several factors, including blood glucose control.

Relationship Between Infertility And Diabetes

Diabetes affects fertility both in males and females. In males, it causes erectile dysfunction by impeding the smooth flow of blood into the spongy tissues of the penis. A man with erectile dysfunction cannot achieve penile penetration of the vagina and

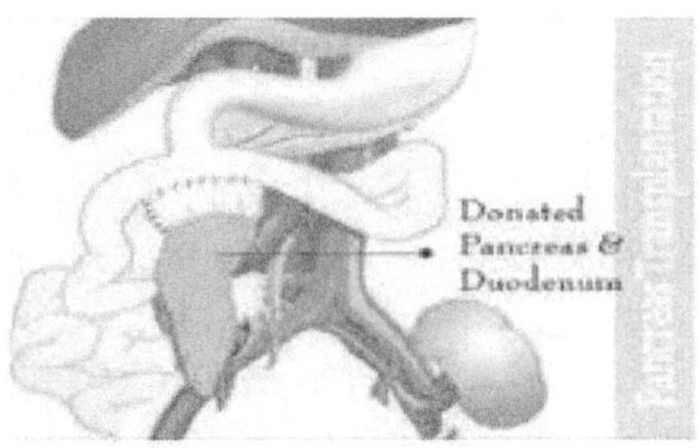

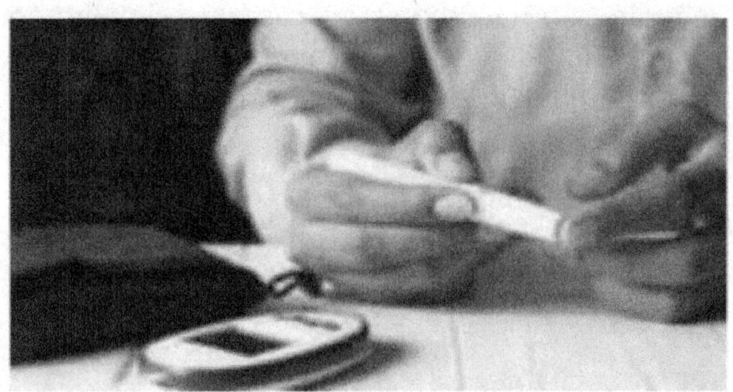

suffers from a weak or un-sustained erection of the penis. These are usually experienced at the advanced stage of Diabetes mellitus.

Can diabetes make it hard for the couple to have a baby?

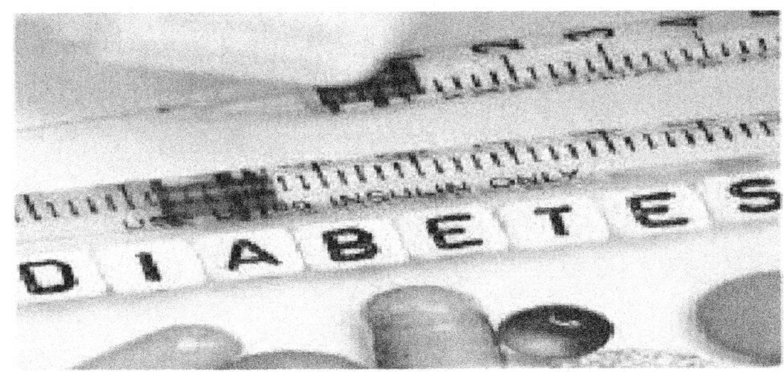

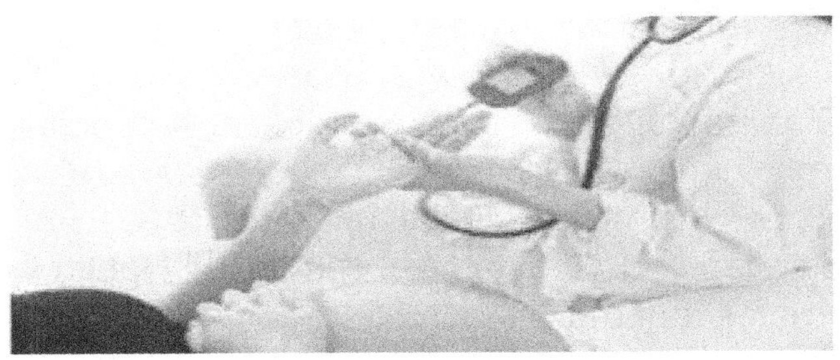

The answer is YES. Diabetes influences your chances of having a baby.

How does diabetes influence fertility?

Diabetes reduces the immunity of the patients. In women where diabetes has reduced the strength of the immune system, the woman becomes prone to various forms of vaginal and other reproductive organ infections. That has a high propensity of making the woman infertile. With severe erectile dysfunction, a man may find it difficult to ejaculate semen into the woman's reproductive tract for natural fertilization.

Diabetes and female infertility

Diabetes mellitus affect your ability to get pregnant and successfully have a baby. Diabetes affects fertility and reproductive health in both men and women. Diabetes can cause hormonal disruptions, resulting in delayed or failed implantation and conception. Diabetes mellitus is associated with poor quality of sperm and embryo and DNA damage, referred to as genetic mutations and deletions. Glucose is an essential source of energy for the body. Usually, glucose requirements and blood glucose levels are well managed by insulin, a glucose-absorbing hormone produced by the pancreas.

When glucose utilization is successfully managed, the body's glucose levels remain in a safe range. Otherwise, the person may experience signs or symptoms of impaired glucose tolerance or diabetes. Diabetes is a condition wherein the pancreas does not make enough insulin as in Type I diabetes, where insulin is not produced. However, if the insulin produced does not work as it should, it is called Type 2 diabetes. The World Health Organization (WHO) estimates that more than 180 million people worldwide have diabetes. Type 1 diabetes is rising alarmingly worldwide, at 3% per annum.

Diabetes and female infertility:

Systematic studies of the metabolic effects of Type 1 Diabetes mellitus (T1DM) and Type 2 Diabetes mellitus (T2DM) on the hypothalamus, pituitary gland, and ovary (HPO) axis have revealed a relationship between these diseases and menstrual disturbances such as delayed menarche or puberty, alterations in the menstrual rhythm including primary and secondary amenorrhea and potential consequences on fertility involving successful conception and fecundity or successful full-term gestation and childbirth.

How diabetes affects fertility

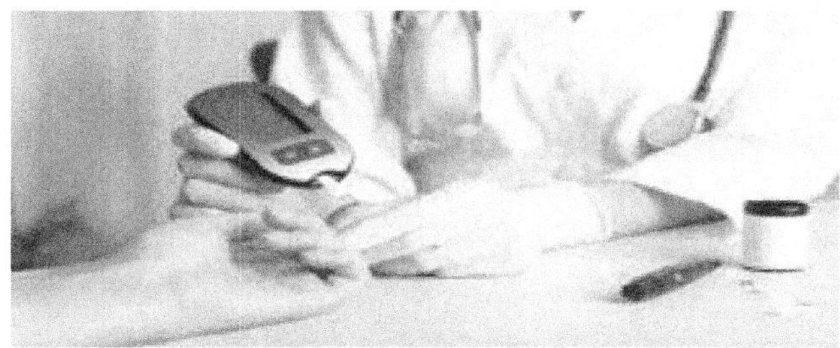

1. Genitourinary infections:

Diabetic women are more susceptible to infection and damage to reproductive organs, especially fallopian tubes. That is due to a reduction in their body immunity, making it easier for pathogenic microbes that have gained entrance into the reproductive tract to thrive. A woman whose immunity has not been compromised by diabetes can fight off these pathogens.

2. Pregnancy complications:

High blood glucose levels can cause miscarriage or congenital disabilities in the fetus: increased blood glucose and excessive nutrition for the growing fetus resulting in macrosomia or big baby syndrome.

3. Decreased libido:

As a result of fatigue or tiredness, depression, and anxiety associated with diabetes, most diabetic women have decreased sexual desire. Also, due to less vaginal

lubrication, women may experience pain and discomfort during sex. That will make them lose interest in sex.

How Type 1 diabetes affects female fertility

1. Menarche and menstrual cycle disturbances:

Type 1 diabetes is associated with longer cycle length,>31 days, and more prolonged menstruation, that is, ≥6 days, heavy menstruation, and menstrual problems at a younger age, <29 years. Juvenile diabetes, as type 1 diabetes, causes delayed menarche.

2. Ovulation:

Ovulation is the absence of ovulation when it would be generally expected, as in a post-menarche and pre-menopausal woman. Ovulation can result from various factors such as chronic mental illness, hormone imbalances, pituitary or ovarian failure, or diabetes. Low BMI diabetic women will have irregular periods, which cause the starving of cells called intracellular starvation. That may disrupt the hypothalamic pulsatile secretion of the gonadotropin-releasing hormone (GnR.H.), which results in a decrease in the secretion of gonadotropins.

Everyone should know that Diabetes mellitus in males and females is associated with infertility. That is to be discussed in the most straightforward language for the benefit of everyone, including those without fundamental knowledge of medically related terms.

An evaluation of the relationship between delayed conception and type 2 diabetes risk, given that there are plausible underlying mechanisms linking the two, including inflammation and insulin resistance, reveals the following:

Persons surveyed included patients free of chronic diseases such as cardiovascular disease, Type 2 diabetes, and cancer at baseline. Empirical evidence on infertility status consisting of>12 months of attempted pregnancy, lifestyle characteristics, and several health-related outcomes has shown a clear correlation between diabetes and infertility. Self-reported cases of diabetes were confirmed using a follow-up questionnaire.

These novel findings suggest a history of infertility, particularly that related to ovulation disorders and tubal blockage, is significantly associated with a higher risk of Type 2 diabetes.

Infertility, commonly defined as failure to achieve pregnancy after more than 12 months of attempting to conceive, affects approximately 12–30% of U.S. couples and higher in West Africa based on estimates from prospective preconception cohorts. Obesity-related metabolic disturbances such as insulin resistance, inflammation, and dyslipidemia have been implicated in some, but not all, infertility-related conditions, particularly ovulatory disorders and polycystic ovary syndrome. Given the common pathologies underlying many causes of infertility and Type 2 diabetes, it is plausible that a history of infertility is related to a risk of diabetes many years later. Evidence suggests a more significant type 2 diabetes risk in women with post-conception obesity syndrome (PCOS).

However, the relationship between other causes of an infertility diagnosis, such as tubal blockages and cervical factors, with subsequent diabetes risk is relatively unexplored.

Few studies have addressed this question prospectively and include careful control for diabetes and possible infertility-related risk. Factors such as body weight and lifestyle. Therefore, the associations of a self-reported history of infertility and its attributed causes with Type 2 diabetes risk in the Nurses" Health Study II (NHS

II) longitudinal cohort of U.S. women have established a strong link between infertility in women and Diabetes mellitus.

The relationship between delayed conception and Type 2 diabetes risk, given that there are plausible underlying mechanisms linking the two, including inflammation and insulin resistance has been evaluated, and the link established. Infertility, commonly defined as failure to achieve pregnancy after more than 12 months of attempting to conceive, affects approximately 12–30% of U.S. couples. Based on estimates from prospective preconception cohorts, this is very prevalent among all reproductive age groups of women but more pronounced in older women.

Obesity-related metabolic disturbances such as insulin resistance, inflammation, and dyslipidemia have been implicated in some, but not all, infertility-related conditions, in particular ovulatory disorders and polycystic ovary syndrome (PCOS). As a result of the common pathologies underlying many causes of infertility and Type 2 diabetes, it is plausible that a history of infertility is related to a risk of diabetes in many people in time to come or simply put as in the recent future.

There is sufficient evidence that suggests a greater type 2 diabetes risk in women with PCOS. However, the relationship between other causes of an infertility diagnosis, such as tubal blockages and cervical factors, culminating in diabetes risk, is relatively unexplored. Other studies have addressed this question and include careful control for diabetes and possible infertility-related risk factors such as body weight and lifestyle. The NHS II is a longitudinal cohort established in 1989 with the enrolment of 116,430 female nurses throughout the USA aged 24–44 years as a baseline. This group is involved in diabetes-related infertility.

Pregnancy loss causes and risk factors

When humans eat, foods are digested in the digestive tract into the simplest elements.

The most straightforward food substances include glucose (a type of sugar belonging to monosaccharides). Glucose is an essential fuel for almost every process in the human body, including brain function. Remember that fuel is any substance, including digested food, burnt to provide energy. For the body to use glucose as energy, it requires a hormone known as insulin, produced by an organ called the pancreas. In diabetes, a person's insulin supply is insufficient or absent, thereby making it impossible for the body to get and use the energy it needs from glucose.

Effects of Diabetes on Pregnancy

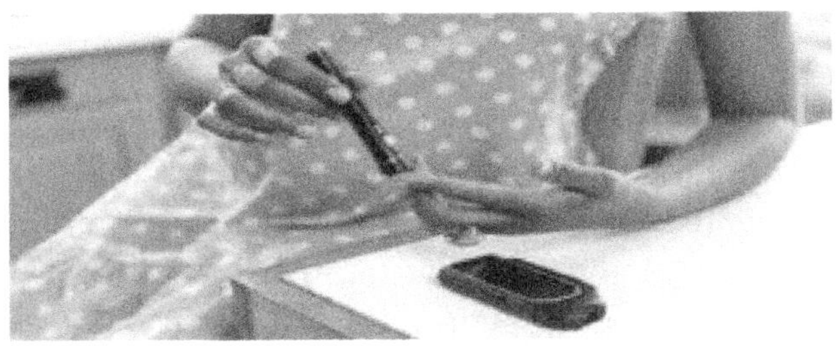

Since the entire body is fueled by glucose, insulin is crucial to the functioning of all body systems. Poorly controlled blood sugar can lead to many complications in pregnancy for both a pregnant woman and her baby.

1. Polyhydramnios:

People with diabetes are more likely to experience having too much amniotic fluid.

2. Hypertension:

It is commonly known as high blood pressure. Hypertension can lead to intrauterine growth restriction (IUGR) and stillbirth and may require pre-term delivery, which carries risks for the baby.

The Link between Diabetes and Miscarriage

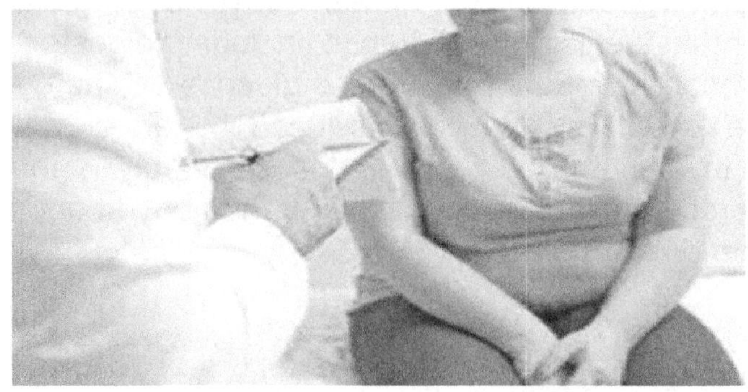

Glucose fuels your body and gives it energy. Virtually every system in your body needs it to function correctly. To turn glucose into energy, you need insulin. Insulin is a hormone produced by the pancreas. When this process breaks down in an individual,

Diabetes mellitus develops. Exercise and a healthy lifestyle are necessary for the effective utilization of insulin by the body.

Type 1 diabetes occurs when your pancreas doesn't produce enough insulin. Type 2 diabetes is when your pancreas produces enough insulin, but your cells have become resistant. A third type, called gestational diabetes, is developed only during pregnancy. It is caused by a disruption in the production and utilization of hormones. All three of these can affect a woman's pregnancy and may lead to miscarriage. Monitoring and managing blood sugar levels during pregnancy are critical. There are health consequences for uncontrolled blood sugar levels in pregnant women. They include

1. Miscarriage

Women with diabetes are at a much greater risk of miscarriage, stillbirth, and neonatal fatalities than women without diabetes. So, suppose you have diabetes and are planning on getting pregnant. It is advisable to control your blood sugar level early to prepare your body for future pregnancy and safe delivery

2. High blood pressure

Hypertension is the medical term for high blood pressure. It is associated with risks even when a woman is not pregnant. However, it could lead to intrauterine growth restriction, preterm delivery, miscarriage, or stillbirth during pregnancy.

3. Increased amniotic fluid

Technically called polyhydramnios, having too much amniotic fluid is another symptom of diabetes. This condition can lead to severe complications, including prolapsed umbilical cord, placental abruption, miscarriage, premature labor, or stillbirth.

4. Post-birth complications

If a pregnant woman avoids a diabetes-related miscarriage, there may still be some complications. Babies born to mothers with uncontrolled diabetes are at higher risk for macrosomia or excess birth weight, which makes delivery difficult. There is also the risk of preterm delivery, which can make feeding and breathing challenging and congenital disabilities of the heart and neural tube.

5. Stillbirth

A pregnant woman can avoid these complications and challenges through medication, nutrition, and careful monitoring.

What to watch for in pregnancy

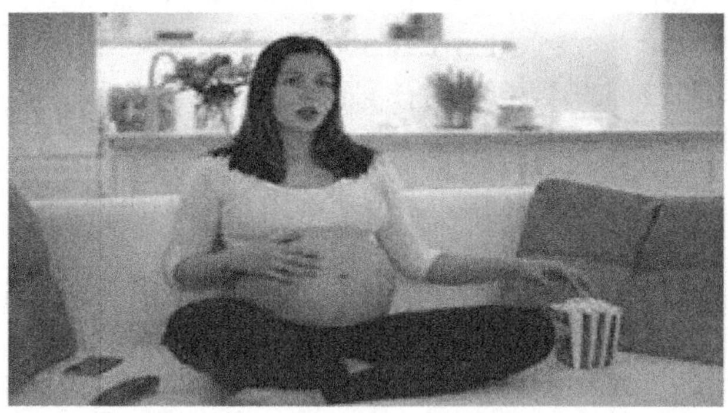

As the pregnancy progresses, a pregnant woman should become her own best health advocate and her baby's first line of defense. Therefore, it is also essential to know the signs of low blood sugar levels. These include:

- ▪ Shaking
- Sweating
- Dizziness
- Racing heart
- Disorientation
- Confusion
- Tingling lips

These are all signs you should expect immediately if you suffer from hypoglycemia or low blood sugar, especially during pregnancy. However, if you feel extremely thirsty, have a dry mouth, and your breath smells fruity, you may have high blood sugar and need medical assistance. You and your baby can make it through a healthy pregnancy despite diabetes if you reduce your blood sugar through healthy lifestyles, diets, and probably medication. Your physician should be of immense assistance to you. Therefore, always consult your physician to guide you.

Talking to Your Partner about Diabetes mellitus Related Fertility Issues

Infertility can be a sensitive subject to talk about, even with your partner. However, if you have been unsuccessfully trying to conceive, it might be time to sit down and discuss your options. Do not panic if you realize that your blood sugar level is below average because stress can exacerbate your situation. The best option is to discuss it with your partner to decide on the best possible option at your disposal to handle the issue. There are many available options that spouses can discuss and adopt to address this issue of diabetes mellitus-induced infertility.

What is involved with IVF?

If you have experienced problems with conception and cannot have a child on your own, In-vitro fertilization (IVF) might be the best option to follow.

Understanding Ovulation

Many women do not pay much attention to their ovulation cycle until they are prepared to get pregnant. You need to know what to do if there are irregular cycles. The best option is to consult your physician. Do not rely on unprofessional advice from unqualified family members and friends whose advice may compound your problem.

Relationship between diabetes and miscarriage during pregnancy

Type 2 diabetes is killing more people than ever, and early-life predictors remain critical for developing effective preventive strategies. Pregnancy loss is a common incidence associated with late rather sclerotic disease and ischaemic heart failure. These may constitute a predictor for type 2 diabetes. This book will enable you to understand whether pregnancy loss is associated with the later development of type 2 Diabetes mellitus or not. That is why the reader should make out time to study this book in detail.

There is a consistent and significant association between pregnancy loss and later Type2 diabetes mellitus increased with an increasing number of losses. Therefore, pregnancy loss and recurrent pregnancy loss is a significant risk factors for later Type 2 Diabetes mellitus. Future studies should explore whether this association is due to common background factors or whether pre-diabetic metabolic conditions are responsible for this association.

The global prevalence of diabetes is 8.5%, and 1.6 million deaths per year are estimated to be directly caused by diabetes. Type 2 diabetes represents 90% of all diabetes. Lifestyle modifications and drug interventions have the potential to prevent Type 2 diabetes which underlines the importance of predictors. Identified predictors for Type 2 diabetes include childhood obesity and gestational diabetes. Predictors for diabetes related to pregnancy are an opportunity to identify women at an increased risk of developing diabetes and to introduce timely preventive actions to nip this in the bud. Regular medical checkups and antenatal clinic attendance are essential to prevent diabetes, hypertension, and eclampsia in pregnant women.

Relationship Between Diabetes Mellitus And Diets In Association With The Lining Mechanisms Type 2 diabetes (T2D) is rapidly growing at an epidemic rate. This epidemic is resulting in increased mortality rates and healthcare costs. Nutrients such as carbohydrates, fat, protein, mineral salts, and vitamins, as well as good disease management, are essential to metabolic homeostasis and therefore present a leading factor contributing to Type 2 diabetes. Therefore, understanding the comprehensive effects and the underlying mechanisms of nutrition in regulating glucose metabolism and the interactions of the diet with genetics, epigenetics, and gut microbiota is essential in developing new strategies to prevent and treat type 2 diabetes (T2D). In this book, I have discussed different mechanistic pathways contributing to T2D and then summarized the current research concerning associations between different nutrient intakes and glucose homeostasis.

I have also explained in this book the possible relationship between nutrients and genetic background, epigenetics, and metagenomics in terms of the susceptibility and treatment of T2D. In some individuals, precision nutrition depends on the person's genotype and microbiota, which are essential in preventing and intervening in T2D.

Diabetes mellitus, considered a disease of minor significance to health, is now becoming one of the main threats to human health both in developed and developing countries (CDC, 20 21). There has been an explosive increase in the number of people diagnosed with diabetes in recent years worldwide. According to the ninth edition of the IDF Diabetes Atlas in 2019, 488 million adults aged 20–99 years are living with diabetes in the world, and the number will reach 578 million by 2030 and 700 million by 2045. It is also projected that 4.2 million adults aged 20–79 years will die of diabetes in the same year. That will account for 11.3% of all deaths, equivalent to eight deaths every minute.

Diabetes is a metabolic disease characterized by persistent hyperglycemia caused by multiple factors, including genetics, nutrition, environment, and physical activity. T2D accounts for more than 90% of all diabetes cases and the diabetes epidemic in the whole world. Insulin resistance and abnormal insulin secretion are the main characteristics of T2D. Apart from the heightened genetic susceptibility of ethnic groups, environment and lifestyles are also very important in the development of T2D.

Globalization, which has resulted in altered dietary and lifestyle habits such as eating more high-fat or high-carbohydrate foods and sedentary lifestyles with low energy expenditure, predisposes individuals to Diabetes mellitus. Diets induce multiple metabolic processes and modify the metabolism homeostasis of the organism. Based on this, unhealthy dietary habits such as high consumption of Western diets by Africans and Asians have been one of the most critical drivers of glucose metabolism disorder that leads to Diabetes mellitus in Africa and, recently, Asia.

The increase in the prevalence of T2D is also associated with the effects of the rise in the incidence of metabolic disorders. Long-term high glucose levels will induce chronic metabolic syndrome, which includes obesity, cardiovascular disease, retinopathy, nephropathy, dyslipidemia, and hypertension. T2D now represents a risk of coronary heart disease, and nearly 80% of diabetic mortality is diabetes-induced cardiovascular disease. The life quality of patients with diabetes decreases due to essentially severe diabetes complications.

Proper diet alone or hypoglycemic agents is the best way to control blood glucose levels in treating T2D. Diets with various nutrient compositions result in changes in metabolites and gut microbiomes that are responsible for the normal glucose metabolism of the whole body because different amino acid content diets can lead to alterations of plasma branched-chain amino acid (BCAA) concentrations. These are linked to the risk of T2D. Fiber and protein-enriched diets change the abundance of Akkermansia muciniphila, thereby decreasing the fasting glucose levels of individuals concerned. However, the interactions between dietary and glucose metabolism need further study to understand the importance of its actions for glucose management.

It is necessary to identify and make suitable dietary solutions that can reduce the prevalence of diabetes and its associated complications. That is achieved by eating different types of food, which constitutes healthy dietary habits. Genome-wide association studies (GWASs) have revealed many genetic variants related to susceptibility to complex diseases. Moreover, the interactions between genetic information and nutrition have recently attracted more attention, as in nutrigenetics. As a result of the genetic variability between individuals, the responses to dietary intakes and utilization vary. Additionally, the specific diet and nutrition modify gene expression, epigenetic features, and a gut microbiome. That calls for more study to understand the pathophysiological mechanisms and precision nutrition solutions to prevent and manage T2D more efficiently.

Therefore, it has become necessary to introduce the significant metabolic pathway related to T2D, such as the insulin signaling pathway, as well as the compounding factors in the morbidity of the disease. However, the roles of macronutrients and other chemicals in maintaining the metabolic homeostasis of the body and their effects on T2D are reviewed in detail.

Additionally, some nutritional recommendations for T2D are summarized based on the perspective of precision nutrition. The diet interactions with genetic background and epigenetic and gut microbiota, which contribute to the risk of T2D, exist in all studies relating diets with blood sugar levels.

The responses to dietary interventions mainly aimed at weight loss and management of insulin resistance are screened for their interaction with genetic and epigenetic features and gut microbiota. These are important in the dietary management of T2D. Therefore, all diabetic patients should take this very seriously for the management of their conditions.

Regulation of Glucose Metabolism

Circulating blood glucose is derived from the diet through intestinal absorption, and the process of glucose production is called gluconeogenesis and glycogen breakdown. Current therapeutic approaches to treat T2D rely on the molecular signaling pathways and targets that impair glucose homeostasis. Therefore, insulin signaling pathway dysregulation of insulin resistance is the main trigger for T2D. Insulin is an endocrine peptide hormone secreted by the pancreas that binds to membrane-bound receptors in target cells of the liver, adipose tissue, and skeletal muscle to trigger metabolic responses to numerous stimuli. Insulin exerts its low glucose function by binding to the insulin receptor (INSR) and then activated INSR recruits phosphor tyrosine binding scaffold proteins such as the INSR substrate (IRS) family. IRS proteins have NH2- terminal pleckstrin homology (P.H.) and PTB domains that target them to activate INSR.

Then, the tyrosine phosphorylates IRS proteins recruit PI3K hetero dimmers that contain a regulatory p85 subunit and a catalytic p110 subunit. PI3K catalyzes the production of phosphatidylinositol-3,4,5- trisphosphate (PIP3) from PIP2 and PIP3 and then recruits proteins with P.H. domains to the plasma membrane, such as pyruvate dehydrogenase kinase 1, which directly phosphorylates AKT. The activated AKT phosphorylates many downstream substrates in various signaling pathways, making it a key node in insulin signaling. The activated insulin signaling reduces glucose production, increases glycogen synthesis, and increases glucose uptake into peripheral tissues such as skeletal muscle and adipose tissue.

In insulin signaling, insulin binds and activates insulin receptors (INSR), causing phosphorylation of insulin receptor substrate (IRS). Tyrosine phosphorylates IRS proteins and recruits phosphatidylinositide-3 (PI3K), which catalyzes the production of phosphatidylinositol-3,4,5- trisphosphate (PIP3) from PIP2. PIP3 then recruits proteins with P.H. domains such as pyruvate dehydrogenase kinase 1 (PDK1), which phosphorylates activating protein kinase B (AKT). These effectors' proteins mediate the effects of insulin on glucose production, utilization, and uptake, as well as glycogen synthesis, which influence the quantity of circulating blood sugar levels. All laypersons could ignore this biochemistry aspect of insulin metabolism in the field of biological sciences because it may sound too academic for easy comprehension by non-biological scientists or medical practitioners.

The dysfunction of insulin signaling will cause insulin resistance. That complex metabolic disorder is closely linked to many pathways, including lipid metabolism, energy expenditure, and inflammation;

hepatic lipid accumulation is known to cause insulin resistance. Diacylglycerol species activate protein kinase C (PKC). This results in impaired insulin signaling. Excess lipid accumulation in the liver is often accompanied by hepatic inflammation. Kupffer cells and macrophages will decrease insulin sensitivity by secreting pro-inflammatory molecules, which activate serine/threonine kinases such as c-Jun N-terminal kinase (JNK) and IκB kinase which in turn impair insulin signaling. Lipid accumulation triggers the unfolded protein response (UPR) pathway.

That impairs insulin signaling. UPR may also alter hepatocyte secretion and contribute to insulin resistance development. Energy expenditure disorder leads to obesity and insulin resistance. That is because non-esterified fatty acids impair β-cell functions, reduce PI3K signaling, and enhance gluconeogenic enzyme expressions. Increased release of tumor necrosis factor α (TNF-α), interleukin 6 (IL6), and monocyte chemotactic protein are responsible for developing insulin resistance.

In addition, hepatocytes which are proteins produced from the liver and secreted into the circulation, play essential roles in regulating insulin signaling also Retinol-binding protein 4(RBP4),α2-macroglobulin (A2M), Fetuin-A (FETUS), fetuin B (FETUB), hepassoc in (FGL1), leukocyte cell-derived chemotaxis 2 (LECT2), and selenoprotein P (SELENOP) are negative regulators of insulin sensitivity. All these substances will cause insulin resistance while fibroblast growth factor 21(FGF21), sex hormone–binding globulin (SHBG), a drop in, and angiopoietin likeprotein4 (ANGPTL4) are positive regulators.

Relationship between lipid metabolism, energy metabolism, inflammation, and insulin resistance

Lipid metabolism and energy metabolism disorders lead to inflammation and affect each other. These are contributory factors to insulin resistance. The mechanisms include diacylglycerol (DAG), activated protein kinase C (PKC), and lipid accumulation which triggers the unfolded protein response (UPR) pathway and results in insulin signaling inhibition; UPR affects hepatocyte secretion to induce insulin resistance. Inflammatory molecules such as tumor necrosis factor α (TNF-α), interleukin 6 (IL6), and monocyte chemotactic protein 1 (MCP1) activate c-Jun N-terminal kinase (JNK) and IκB kinase (IKK), which subsequently impair insulin signaling; energy homeostasis disorder and β- cell functions which reduce PI3K signaling and facilitates gluconeogenic enzyme expressions and later causing insulin resistance. Insulin resistance is a principal cause of diabetes in human beings.

Carbohydrate

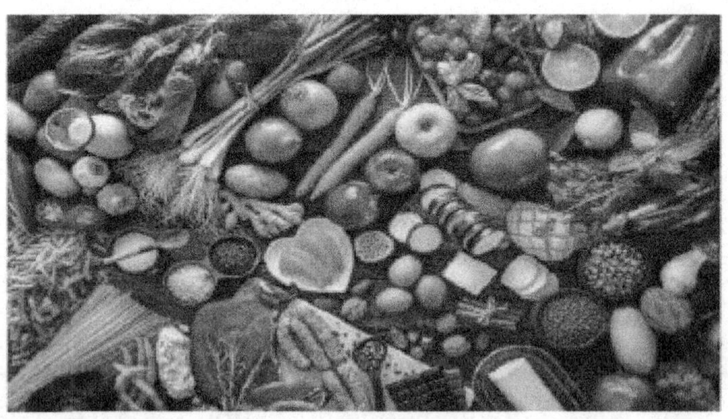

It requires precise control of glucose metabolism to maintain metabolic homeostasis in the body. Hormonal regulation and the associated enzyme transcription induced by various. In response to glucose availability, Metabolites are mainly responsible for this control mechanism. Insulin triggers INSR auto-phosphorylation, then recruits and phosphorylates I.R. substrates 1 and 2 (IRS1/2), resulting in phosphatidylinositide-3, 4, 5-P3 (PIP3) production. That activates protein kinase B (PKB/AKT).

Therefore, it promotes glucose uptake by different tissues and organs, including the liver, adipose tissue, and skeletal muscle. It inhibits hepatic glucose output and increases glycogen synthesis. However, it also decreases glycogen decomposition. Insulin triggers off anabolic responses such as ribosome biogenesis and protein synthesis. All these are dependent on the nutritional state of individuals. The TOR/S6K1 signaling pathway is also activated by insulin and plays a vital role in regulating glucose homeostasis. Glucose released by diet, therefore, stimulates the production of PI3P, recruiting proteins to the membranes of the endosome and subsequently activating mTOR/S6K1, which signals glucose homeostasis.

Glucose homeostasis involves different pathways, carried out partly by the transcriptional control of related genes. Carbohydrate triggers the expressions of enzymes, including pyruvate kinase, glucokinase, ATP citrate lyase, and acetyl CoA carboxylase. These genes are regulated by the carbohydrate-responsive element-binding protein (ChREBP), which is a helix–loop–helix leucine, a zipper transcription factor. Also, it plays a very significant role in sugar-induced lipogenesis and glucose homeostasis. It does this by regulating carbohydrate digestion and transport. In responding to the glucose, ChREBP forms a hetero dimer and activates the target gene transcriptions, which contain five carbohydrate response element motifs. Besides its glucose sensor role, ChREBP is also essential for fructose-induced lipogenesis in the liver and intestine, possibly through the ChREBP-FGF21 signaling axis.

The role of nutrients in T2D

Carbohydrates regulate glucose homeostasis through carbohydrate-responsive element-binding protein (ChREBP) induced glucose metabolism-related gene expressions. Fatty acids inhibit AKT/PKB activation and impair the insulin signaling pathway. Apart from that, the fat causes reactive oxygen species (ROS) generation in mitochondria and activates peroxisome proliferators-activated receptors (PPARs), which collectively mediate the regulation of fat on glucose metabolism. The possible pathways or mechanisms of protein/amino acids affecting glucose levels include insulin secretion, glucose uptake, hormone release, mTOR/S6K1 signaling pathway, and GCN2/eIF2α/ATF4 transduction pathway. Mineral substances activate cofactors and coenzymes for metabolism control, oxidative stress, and genetic transcription. It makes them play roles in glucose transport and redox reactions and affects glucose homeostasis. Vitamin has a role in regulating glucose utilization, insulin signaling, and insulin release from β cells to maintain blood glucose levels. It is also the modulator of inflammatory cytokines related to glucose metabolism.

Carbohydrate foods that promote sustained but low glucose levels may benefit metabolic control of diabetes and its complications. Fiber-rich food serves this purpose. Diets with slow-release carbohydrates lower the glucose and insulin responses throughout the day and improve the capacity for fibrinolysis. It may be a potential therapy for T2D. When syrup is included in a diabetic diet, it is better to consider sucrose instead of fructose. In a short-term trial of T2D patients in the United States of America, scientists showed that iso-caloric fructose replacement of other carbohydrates such as sucrose and starch improved glycemia control and had no effects on insulin signaling. However, it should be considered that high sucrose or fructose diet is not recommended for diabetic individuals and others with impaired glucose metabolism. Sucrose is a disaccharide that digests faster than a polysaccharide such as starch. Apart from this, specific diet components may affect the regulatory role of foods on blood glucose levels.

A diet with fiber, some proteins, or lipids mixed may influence the rates of carbohydrate digestion and absorption. It may be beneficial to T2D patients. Polyols have been used as sugar replacers for almost a century. A clinical trial showed that polyols had a role in lowering serum glucose levels in T2D patients. It may provide a new strategy for managing T2D.

Dietary fibers mainly found in cereals, fruits, vegetables, or legumes have been closely associated with T2D. They are essential in helping to reduce blood glucose levels. While increased fiber intake, particularly soluble fibers, is known to play beneficial roles in improving glycaemic control in patients with T2D, low fiber-containing diets such as white bread and refined sugars do the contrary. Therefore, white bread and refined sugars should be avoided by patients suffering from Diabetes mellitus for effective management.

Fats and Oil

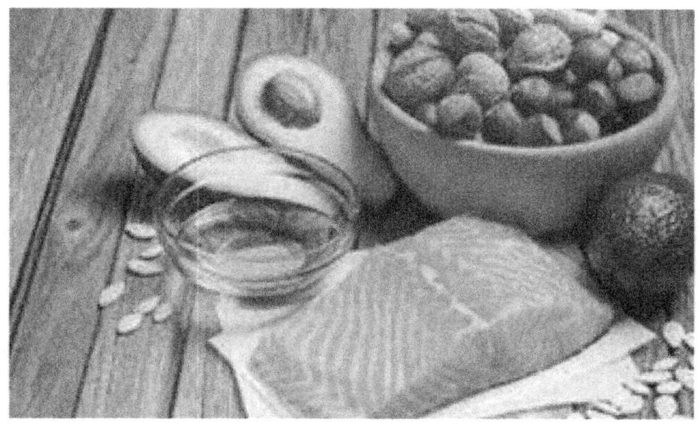

These are collectively called lipids. Lipid in liquid form is referred to as oil, while lipid in solid form is known as fat. Lipids are both dangerous and beneficial in the formation of cell membranes. The high-density lipids (HDLs) are suitable because they do not constitute many health problems, unlike the low-density lipids.

Our body obtains lipid metabolites from diet intake directly or generated intra-cellular by the liver and fatty tissues in multiple pathways. Lipidomics helps us to understand the circulating lipid species better. Some are considered biomarkers that are related to insulin resistance.

They include stearic acid, deoxy sphingoid lipids, and saturation and chain length of fatty acids. High-fat diet-induced insulin resistance and T2D have been primarily known for two decades. A high-fat diet increases lipid accumulation in cells and results in obesity, and excess fat increases pro-inflammatory cytokines and other hormones or factors responsible for insulin resistance.

Free fatty acids inhibit Akt/PKB activation, impairing the insulin signaling pathway. Apart from this, the reactive oxygen species generation in mitochondria is increased. It also affects glucose homeostasis. Peroxisome proliferator-activated receptors (PPARs) function as lipid sensors that can activate dietary fatty acids and their derivatives. PPARs regulate the expression of genes involved in various processes, such as glucose and lipid metabolism, immune response, and cell growth. PPARα is essential in regulating fatty acid oxidation, and so has indirect effects on improving glucose metabolism. However, PPARα activates tribbles pseudokinase 3 (TRB3), a direct target, to inhibit AKT activation and impair insulin sensitivity. PPARγ is an effector of adipogenesis through C/EBP responsible for glucose regulation.

The impact of fatty acid intake on blood glucose and insulin in the diet of adults with T2D has shown that replacing saturated fats with monounsaturated fatty acids (MUFAs) or polyunsaturated fatty acids may improve their glucose or insulin tolerance. In-vitro experiments have confirmed that MUFAs or oleate rather than palmitate prevents insulin resistance. Recent studies have shown that postprandial hyperlipidemia is common in T2D patients and that omega-3 fatty acids could reduce postprandial lipids but may not correct them completely. The role of transfats in regulating glucose control is still controversial. Meta-analysis has shown that a cholesterol-rich diet positively correlates with T2D risk. Additionally, supplementation of plant sterols or stanols lowers serum cholesterol levels, which may indirectly benefit glucose metabolism.

Protein

Dietary proteins are vital to life because of their significant role in acquiring essential amino acids to maintain protein synthesis and degradation and supporting cellular processes such as cell growth and development. More intensive studies have shown that proteins affect glucose homeostasis differently by affecting insulin action and secretion, except for body weight and feeding behavior. Dietary proteins stimulate insulin secretion in normal or diabetic patients to reduce glycemia. Highprotein diets appear to have beneficial effects on weight loss and glucose metabolism, increase insulin sensitivity and decrease inflammation in the short term. However, long-term high-protein intake seems to lead to insulin resistance in the whole body; This is possible by increasing the mTOR/S6K1 signaling pathway and stimulating gluconeogenesis and high glucagon turnover.

Studies have shown that a 6-month high-protein diet (1.87 ± 0.26 g protein/kg body weight per day) in healthy individuals increases fasting glucose levels, impaired hepatic glucose output suppression by insulin, and enhanced gluconeogenesis. On the other hand, low-protein diets consisting of 5%–10% protein calories suggest improved insulin sensitivity that is beneficial to T2D. It may be achieved through the general control non-de repressible 2 (GCN2)/transcription factor 4 (ATF4)/FGF21 signaling pathway. Protein from the soya bean is a type of protein suitable for its hypo-lipidemic and hypocholesterolemic benefits in diabetic patients.

Studies have shown that soy protein intake can positively affect glucose metabolism and decrease serum lipids. Compared with casein, reduces fasting glucose and insulin levels in animals and prevents insulin resistance induced by a high-sucrose diet. However, in humans, it has been revealed that soy protein decreases glucose levels compared to casein.

The differential hormonal response might explain this function. Also, soy protein can stimulate INSR mRNA expression and increase insulin signaling in fat and liver, thereby improving insulin sensitivity in these tissues and organs.

Fish protein is a first-class protein and has been widely known for years in the United States of America's Alaska and Greenland populations, with a low incidence of T2D for taking large amounts of fish. In lean fish, protein is the most abundant nutrient source. Therefore, fish protein consumption shows improved cholesterol transport through high-density lipoprotein and reduced triglycerides, thus very low-density lipoprotein. However, compared with casein-fed animals, cod protein–fed rats can be protected from insulin resistance-induced Diabetes by sucrose or saturated fat through stimulating glucose uptake by skeletal muscle. Also, a cod protein activated PI3K/AKT signaling pathway and selectively improved GLUT4 translocation to the T tubules, thereby improving glucose transport in response to insulin. Moreover, human studies have shown that cod protein exerts many beneficial effects on T2D. Cod protein induces a lower insulin-to-glucose ratio compared with milk protein and increased post-meal plasma insulin concentrations compared with beef protein. Protein breakdown or synthesis leads to a change in amino acid levels.

We have eight amino acids that cannot be produced inside the body but are derived from food. These are essential amino acids. Amino acids are considered gene expression regulators. A healthy and balanced diet should meet all the requirements in amino acids and proteins from various sources of food substances in their proper proportions. When there is a decrease in essential amino acids, it causes the de- acetylation of the corresponding transfer ribonucleic acids (tRNAs). Neutral tRNAs bind and activate the GCN2 kinase, and subsequently, the activated GCN2 phosphorylates the eukaryotic initiation factor 2α (eIF2α) and induces Wellington 365 81 ATF4 activation. Recent studies have shown that increasing dietary levels of BCAAs had a positive effect on T2D. There are suggestions that deficiency of BCAAs was beneficial for improving insulin sensitivity and glucose tolerance. Leucine deprivation or methionine deficiency shows improved insulin sensitivity, energy expenditure, and thermogenesis through the GCN2/eIF2α/ATF4/FGF21 transduction pathway.

Micronutrients and T2D as micronutrients or mineral substances are required at low concentrations for normal body metabolism; they play significant roles in maintaining metabolism homeostasis. Some mineral substances activate cofactors and coenzymes for metabolism control, oxidative stress, and genetic transcription. The deficiency of mineral substances has been shown to have a relationship with T2D. Selenium is an essential component of enzymes for redox reactions, such as glutathione peroxidase and thioredoxin reductase in humans. The dose range to toxicity is very slim. The primary dietary sources of selenium are cereals, black tea, milk, mushrooms, soybeans, bamboo shoots, nuts, broccoli, cassava leaves, and spinach. The average concentration of selenium intake can act as insulin mimetics to attenuate Diabetes, thereby decreasing glucose and insulin tolerance.

It prevents hepatic insulin resistance. High selenium concentration will lead to gluconeogenesis, and fasting blood glucose (FBG) levels will increase, resulting in diabetes complications. Vanadium is standard but appears at low concentrations in humans. It occurs with proteins such as transferrin, albumin, and hemoglobin. These are vital to the physiological processes in humans. In-vitro and in-vivo researches suggest that vanadium has insulin-mimetic properties that may be a potential therapeutic agent for T2D. Oral administration of 1 mg/kg daily of vanadyl sulfate for 4 weeks significantly decreases glucose levels in diabetes patients. It might be possible through a mechanism underlying this by increasing GLUT translocation to the plasma membrane, which subsequently increases glucose transport.

Chromium plays a prominent role in glucose metabolism by facilitating insulin binding to INSR. Chromium supplements significantly decrease postprandial and also fasting glucose levels. Mechanisms for this beneficial function of chromium may partly be adduced to the increase of GLUT2 expression and the activation of the PI3K/AKT pathway in skeletal muscle. Zinc is an essential component of enzymes that play vital roles in regulating insulin sensitivity and glucose homeostasis. Researchers have shown that, in patients with T2D, the concentrations of zinc in plasma and tissues are lower. Zinc supplements improve insulin sensitivity and glucose tolerance in experimental diabetic mice models. It has also been found to have similar functions in humans.

High sodium intake results in a higher risk of hypertension and cardiovascular diseases in patients with Diabetes mellitus. Excess sodium intake increases natriuresis through PPARδ/SGLT2 pathway and subsequently regulates glucose metabolism of Type 2 diabetic patients. In contrast, another magnesium substance decreases the risk of cardiovascular diseases in T2D patients. Magnesium deficiency is associated with diabetes risk, while magnesium supplementation could attenuate insulin resistance and improve glycaemic control in T2D patients.

Vitamin

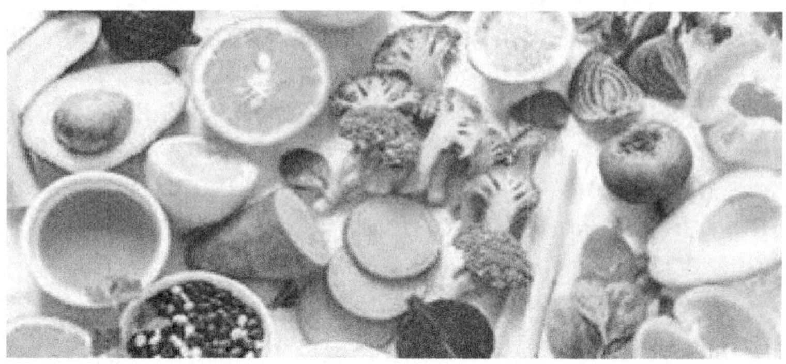

Recently, the vitamin has received increased attention due to its role in regulating the development of T2D by modulating insulin resistance and pancreatic β-cell functions. Also, vitamins D and E are the two most popular vitamins in regulating blood glucose levels. Vitamin D is used to regulate bone metabolism but is found to have various clinical functions, such as acting as a catalyst for producing the hormone involved in calcium and phosphorus balance. Vitamin D receptor (VDR) is found in the pancreatic β cells and insulin response tissues such as skeletal muscle and adipose tissues. Recent studies have shown that vitamin D affected glucose utilization in a VDR- dependent manner in muscles and adipose tissues and activated PPARδ, a transcription factor involved in fatty acid metabolism. Besides that, vitamins modulated insulin action and sensitivity by directly stimulating INSR gene expressions or altered calcium flux to influence the insulin release of β cells. However, the vitamin is a negative modulator of inflammatory cytokines such as

TNF-α and IL6, closely related to insulin resistance. Insulin resistance is the primary diagnosis in most T2D patients. Vitamin D deficiency has resulted in insulin resistance and metabolic syndrome, including hypo- gonadotrophic, renal diseases, and cardiovascular complications.

Some beneficial effects of vitamin D supplements have been reported. Several clinical trials have shown that vitamin D administration decreases serum fasting glucose levels and improves homeostatic model assessment of insulin resistance index in T2D patients. Vitamine is a fat-soluble vitamin known for its antioxidant capacity in humans. For some time now, vitamin E has been reported to have a role in regulating insulin sensitivity. Vitamin E supplements significantly decrease plasma glucose and hemoglobin A1c (HbA1c) levels. The underlying mechanisms may involve several pathways, including antioxidant capacity. Vitamin E alters IRS1 phosphorylation, thereby affecting insulin signaling. Besides, vitamin E is known to directly regulate gene expression, such as PPARγ, which plays significant and active roles in insulin sensitivity.

Other Chemicals and T2D

Besides macronutrients and micronutrients, other factors such as phytochemicals and bio-actives widely distributed in diets or chemicals (such as alcohol) also have potential effects on T2D. Phytochemicals or bio-actives exist in herbaceous plant species' fruits, flowers, wood, seeds, bark, and stems. However, some of them are found in traditional Chinese medicines. Their beneficial and therapeutic roles in diabetes in various studies have been studied and elucidated. Phytochemical compounds, which include lignin or flavonoids, protect the body from oxidative stress and help diabetic wound healing. Bio- actives, such as curcumin, capsaicin, berberine, cilantro, or artemisinin, has shown to improve insulin sensitivity to combat diabetes.

Despite these immense benefits, the biomolecular activity and toxicity of these phytochemicals and bio-actives need to be studied further. It will help to understand their mechanisms for enhancing insulin sensitivity. Alcohol is closely related to diseases such as fatty liver, cardiovascular diseases, and T2D. A dose-response meta-analysis suggests that light and moderate alcohol intake may reduce the risk of T2D, whereas heavy alcohol intake shows an inconclusive association. Nutritional recommendations for T2D Clinical trials suggest different nutritional recommendations for preventing and managing T2D, and they all emphasize the importance of dietary habits and lifestyles. Calorie restriction and exercise help reduce the risk of T2D through weight loss.

Based on this perspective of nutrients, quality is more important than quantity. For improving glucose control in T2D patients, diets rich in fruits, vegetables, legumes, and whole grains are recommended. Low-carbohydrate, low-GI (glycemic index), and high-protein diet patterns will protect us from hyperglycemia. Moderate consumption of nuts and alcohol is also beneficial in reducing blood glucose levels. Various populations or individuals have different foods, dietary habits, and disease susceptibility, so nutritional strategies have to vary according to their cultures and genetic backgrounds.

A diet with Genetics, Epigenetics, and Metagenomics Involved in the Risk of T2D Genetic backgrounds and environments, such as high-fat and high-energy dietary habits and a sedentary lifestyle, are significant factors that contribute to the high susceptibility of T2D. Recent advances in precision nutrition have recognized that an individual's diet may increase the risk of T2D by interacting with specific gene variants that affect the expression of genes, modifying the epigenetic features, or altering microbial composition involved in critical metabolic pathways.

The relationship between diabetes and economic development

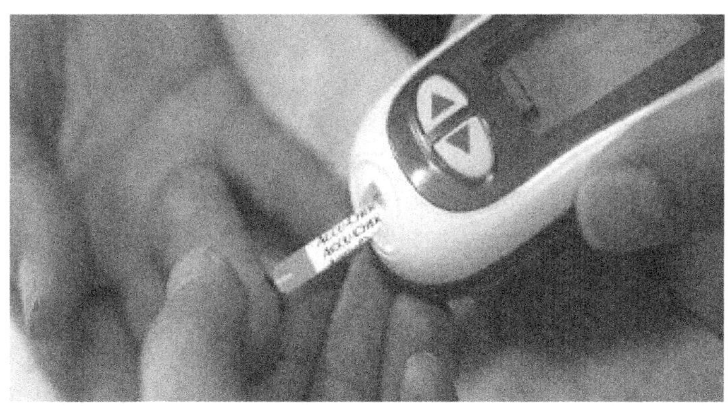

Diabetes mellitus is a disorder caused by insufficient or insufficient production of the pancreas's hormone called insulin. The World Health Organization (WHO) estimates that more than 180 million people globally have Diabetes. An estimated 2.9 million people died from Diabetes, that is, a case-fatality rate (CFR) of 0.0161. In 2000, the prevalence of Diabetes in the African Region was estimated at 7.02 million people, of which about 0.702 million (10%) people had type 1 diabetes, and 6.318 million (90%) had type 2 diabetes. Approximately 113,100 people died from diabetes-related causes, 561,600 were permanently disabled, and 6,458,400 experienced temporary disability.

Diabetes exerts a heavy economic burden on every community and country. This burden is related to health system costs incurred by various countries in managing and treating the disease. Indirect costs are resulting from productivity losses due to patient disability and premature death and time spent by family members accompanying patients when seeking care. However, intangible costs cause financial and time loss to the individuals or organizations concerned. There is also an associated psychological pain to the family and friends.

It is estimated that the total annual costs associated with Diabetes in Latin America and the Caribbean are US$65.216 billion. The direct price is US$10.721 billion, and the indirect cost is US$54.495 billion. It is estimated that with a conservative prevalence of 200,000 type 1 diabetic subjects in India, the cost of treatment could be as high as US$50 million. The American Diabetes Association estimated that the combined direct and indirect costs of Diabetes in 1997 were US$98 billion in the United States of America. It is estimated that the total direct costs of Diabetes are over US$650 million in Spain, where there were over 1.4 million known diabetics in 1994 and the cost of type 1 diabetes in England and Wales is US$1.92 million or US$2042 per person. Unfortunately, there is a pool of similar evidence for the African Region. Generally, there is global ascendency in cases of Diabetes mellitus with a corresponding increase in the cost of management and treatment. Changes in lifestyles may account for these phenomena.

This book focuses on the economic burden of Diabetes in the African Region and other regions, including America, Europe, and Asia. It attempts to answer questions: from a societal perspective, specifically the ministries of health and the families, what is the total cost of Diabetes to the Regions? The specific objectives were to estimate the direct costs that are borne by the health systems and the families in directly addressing the problems and the indirect costs, that is., the losses in productivity attributable to premature mortality, permanent disability, and temporary disability associated with Diabetes mellitus.

One of the significant threats to economic development confronting the 53 Member States of the African countries is the growing burden of Diabetes and other non-communicable diseases. The effectiveness of prevention and control of those diseases hinges mainly on the health system's performance of its functions of leadership and governance; health workforce; Medical products, vaccines, and technologies, information, financing, and services delivery. In the Region, the total numbers of physicians are 2,281,643; nurses are3,383,925; midwives are 111,895; dentists are 506,898; pharmacists are 518,378; public and environmental health workers are 177,887; community health workers are 163,285; laboratory technicians are 274,011; other health workers are1,361,467 and health management and support workers are 2,521,510.

The physician density per 1000 was 0.03–0.78 in 18 countries; 1.01–2.00 in 14 countries, 2.14–3.00 in 4 countries, 3.01–4.00 in 7 countries, and over 4.00 in 3 countries. The nurse Density per 1000 was 0.14–0.96 in 17 countries, 1.05–2.00 in 4 countries, 2.10–3.00 in 4 Countries, 3.01–4.00 in 8 countries, and over 4.00 in 13 countries. Laboratory technician density varied from a minimum of 0.01 per 1000 in Niger to a maximum of 0.65 per 1000 in Côte D'Ivoire. Sixty-three percent of the 57 countries experiencing extreme shortages of health workers worldwide are in the African Region. The scarcity of qualified health workers impacts the effective management of Diabetes mellitus negatively. About 50% of the population in the Region lacks access to essential medicines. The number of hospital beds per 100000 persons among 33 countries that had data was as follows: 8(24%) countries had 3–20 beds, 13 (39%) countries had 21– 40 beds, and 12 (36%) countries had more than 40 beds per 100000.

In 2005, the per capita total expenditure on health in purchasing power parity international dollars (PPP Int$) was $30 and less in 6 countries; $31–60 in 14 countries; $61–90 in 8 countries, $91–120 in 4 countries; and $122–811 in 14 countries. General government expenditure on health as a percentage of total expenditure was 30% and less in 7 countries; 31–50% in 13 countries; 51–70% in 17 countries; and 71–90% in 9 countries.

The health systems challenges allude to the above statistics regarding the situation where 47% of the population in the Region has no access to quality health services. Those health systems bottlenecks also hamper effective responses to the growing burden of Diabetes and other noncommunicable diseases.

The distribution by age of Diabetes mellitus was used to disaggregate the total number of people with Diabetes into age groups in Africa. The gross national income (GNI) per capita in purchasing power parity (PPP) was obtained from the World Bank and calculated. The implied PPP conversion rates used in converting national currencies into current international dollars were from an

International Monetary Fund website. The prices of diabetes medicines were obtained from a WHO/AFRO publication, and the hotel component of hospital costs, excluding drugs and diagnostic tests, were obtained from a WHO website. The 46 member states in the WHO African Region were classified into three groups using gross national income (GNI) per capita expressed in purchasing power parity for 2005.

Classification of countries according to gross national income per capita, PPP 2005 international dollars in 2005 the direct costs related to the treatment of diabetes patients were obtained from various sources from one or more countries in each group. Each group's average cost figure for various health system inputs and GNI was obtained and used in the analysis. The different countries' costs of other information used in the treatment of Diabetes were converted into current international dollar equivalents using PPP conversion rates to ensure that prices of different inputs were similar in each country group. An example is the Mauritian Lipid test cost of Int$28.9 was obtained by dividing the local cost for Lipid profile test R424 by the implied PPP conversion rate of 14.677. A discount rate of 3%was used to convert future indirect price flows into their present values (WHO diabetes program, 2008)). Definition of costs estimated.

The economic burden of Diabetes comprises direct costs, indirect costs, and intangible costs. The direct cost has two components. Firstly, the prices of organizing and operating hospital services which include hotel costs under human resources-for-health time, utilities, food, nonpharmaceutical supplies, diagnostic equipment, building space, diagnostic tests such as HBA1c test, lipid profile, proteinuria test, blood sugar test, electrocardiogram, medicines such as insulin, oral drugs, and devices for injecting insulin or simply syringes. Secondly, the patients and their families bear out-of-pocket expenses, including health service provider consultation fees, medicines, tests, and transport. All these form the costs of management and treatment of Diabetes mellitus in Africa, where poverty and underdevelopment are still rife.

The indirect costs involve all the opportunity costs of time lost due to morbidity emanating from a temporary disability, permanent disability, and premature mortality. The morbidity-related component includes the productivity losses of time invested by patients in outpatient department (OPD) consultations, travel to and from hospitals, waiting for admission, As well as during institutionalized treatment; by relatives who accompany patients during pre-admission talks, travel to and from hospitals attending patients, waiting for patients to be admitted, and visiting patients after admission. The premature mortality-related cost component is equal to the lost work years due to sudden death calculated using: retirement age minus age at death multiplied by average remuneration per year. Intangible costs are welfare losses due to physical and psychological pain. Consequent to the stigma attached to chronic diseases, the related psychic and social costs to the affected families can be profound. The intangible costs were calculated to appreciate the financial burden of Diabetes mellitus fully.

Analytical model

The total cost (TC) incurred by ministries of health, diabetes patients, and family members can be expressed as follows: TC=DC+ IC+ ITC Where: DC is the direct cost; IC is an indirect cost which is the value of productivity multiplied by time lost.ITC is an intangible cost, including physical and psychological pain

Direct costs

The total direct costs (DC) were estimated using the following variables and equations: DC=TCI+TCS+TCR +TCM+TCD +TCOC+TCH +TCT +OoPE Where: TCI is the total annual cost of insulin; TCS is the yearly total cost of syringes; TCR is the total annual cost of reagent strips; TCM is the total yearly cost of glucometer; TCD is the total cost of oral drugs; TCOC is the total cost of OPD consultations; TCH is the total cost of hospitalization; TCT is the total cost of Diabetes related test for all people with Diabetes;

and OoPE is the out-of-pocket expenses borne by patients, family members, and relatives.

Insulin

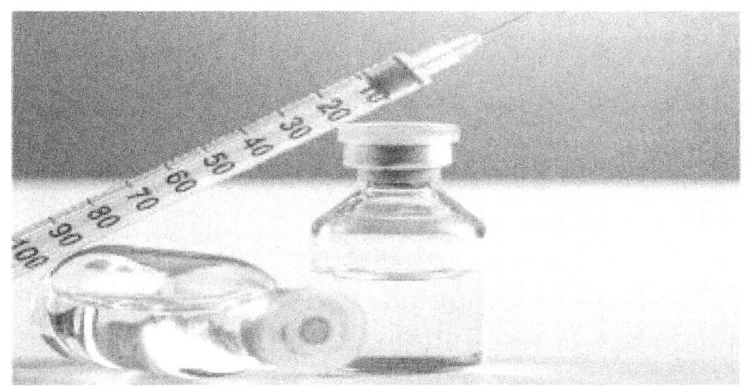

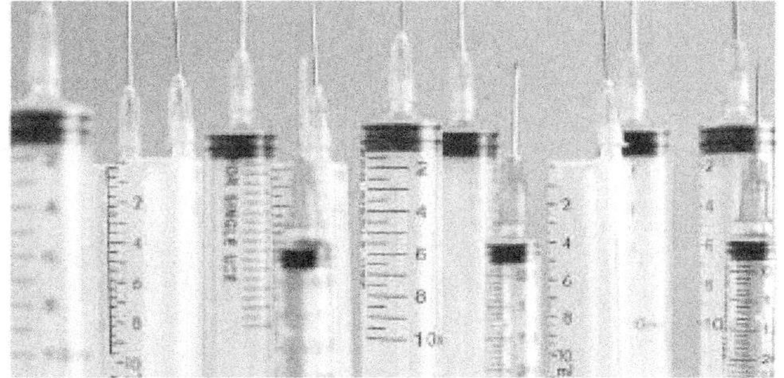

Syringes

The total annual cost of insulin for n the group of countries (TCI n) was estimated using the following formula: TCI n = (NII n × AQP × P in); where: NII n is the total number of patients in need of insulin, which is equal to all the type 1 diabetes patients plus 5% of the type2 diabetes patients; AQP is the annual quantity of insulin consumed per patient per year, that is. 10000 IU; P in is the average price per unit of insulin expressed in international dollars for n is the group of countries.

The annual cost of syringes for the nth group of countries (TCS) was obtained as follows:

TCS n = NII n × DIY × P sn; where: DIY is the number of days in a year and P in is the average price per unit of syringe expressed in international dollars for the nth group of countries.

Reagent strips

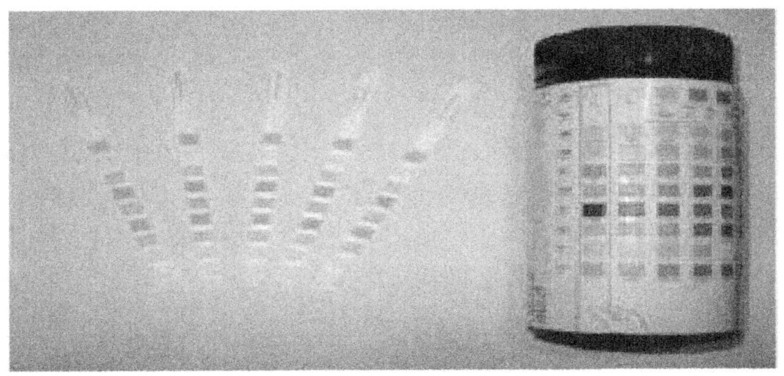

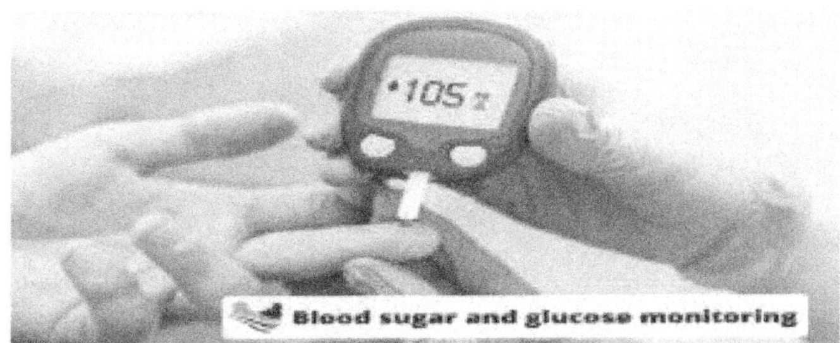

Glucose meters (Glycometer)

The annual cost of **reagent strips** for the nth group of countries (TCRn) was obtained as follows: TCSn= NIIn × TRSU × DIY × PRSn; where: TRSU is the number of times a reagent strip is used in a day, DIY is the number of days in a year and P RSS is the average price per unit of reagent strip expressed in international dollars for the nth group of countries.

The annual cost of **glucose meters** for the nth group of countries (TCM n) was derived as follows: TCM n = [(AC n × QGM n)/A(0.03,5)]; where: QGM n is the number of glucose meters needed, that is equal to the number of insulin users; AC n is the annual equivalent cost of one glucose meter in international dollars for an nth group of countries, and A(5,0.03) is the annuity factor calculated assuming a 5-year useful life and a 3% discount rate. The annuity factor was obtained using the following formula: For example, dividing the Group 1 countries' average replacement cost of Int$30.97 per glucose meter by the annuity factor yields an annual equivalent cost of 30.97/4.579707 = Int$6.762441.

Oral drugs

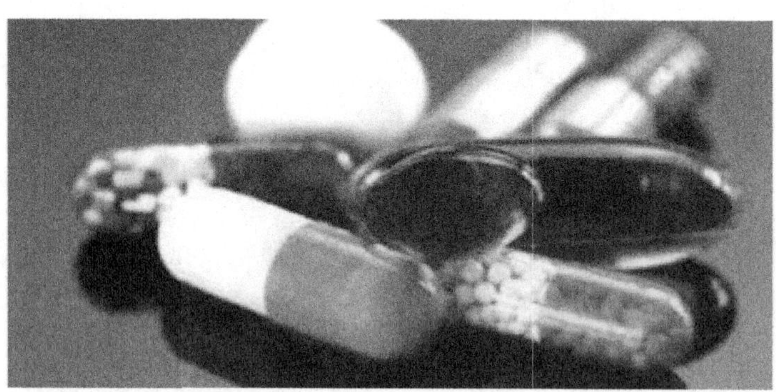

The annual total cost of oral drugs for the nth group of countries (TCD n) was calculated as follows: TCD n = NOD n × NTY × P Mn; NOD n is the total number of people in need of oral drugs in the nth group of countries; NTY is the number of 500 mg Metformin tablets taken per person per year, and P Mn is the average PPP price per 500 mg Metformin tablet in an nth group of countries. In our estimation of the TCD, we assumed that 80% of the total population with type 2 diabetes in each group of countries will need oral drugs and the total number of Metformin tablets needed per person per year would be 1500 (World Bank data and research, 2008).

Outpatient consultations and hospitalizations

The hospital cost per hospital stay and outpatient visit represent only the hotel component, excluding drugs and diagnostic tests and other costs such as personnel, capital, and food costs. The hotel component of the hospital costs was obtained from a WHO website. The cost of hospital outpatient department consultations (TCOC n) was calculated as follows: TCOC n = ND n × NV × CV n; where: ND n is the total number of diabetics in an nth group of countries; NV is the total number of OPD visits by a diabetes patient per year in an nth group of countries, and CV n is the cost per OPD visit in international dollars in an nth group of countries. An example is the TCOC for group 1 countries where NB = 974000, NV = 4, CV n = Int$39.95 was 974000 × 4 × 39.9483333333333 = Int$155638707.

The total cost of diabetes patient hospitalizations per year in an nth group of countries (CHOPn) was calculated as follows:

CHOPn= NHPn × ALSn × CPIDn

Where: NHP is the total number of patients hospitalized (Type 1 + 5% of Type 2), ALS is the average length of stay, and CPID is the cost per inpatient day. It is assumed that all people with diabetes will make four visits a year to a hospital outpatient department. In addition, we assumed that all patients with Type1 diabetes plus 5% of patients with Type2 diabetes would require one hospitalization per year and that the average length of stay for diabetes patients is 9 days. For instance, the TCOC for group 1 countries (NHP= 146100, ALS= 9.08CPID= Int$91.10) was 146100 × 9.07979554747842 × 91.1008333333333 = Int$120850551.

Tests

The total cost of diabetes-related tests [4] for the nth group of countries (TCT) was estimated as follows:

TCTn= (NDN)×(CHBAn+CLP n+CECGn+CPTn+CBSn);

Where: ND n is the total number of people with diabetes; CHBA n is the cost of one HBA1c test; CLP n is the cost of one lipid profile; CECG n is the cost of one electrocardiogram; CPT n is the cost of one protein urea test, and CBS n is the cost of one blood sugar test. We estimated that, in a year, a total of all the 7.02 million people with diabetes would require one HBA1c test, one lipid profile test, one proteinuria test, and one electrocardiogram. The average cost of these tests for Group 1 countries was obtained by WHO Country Offices health systems staff from Mauritius; Group 2 from Congo, Namibia, and Swaziland; and Group 3 from Kenya, Mauritania, and Senegal. From calculations of TCT using group 1 data:

ND = 974000; CHBA=Int$24.77368051; CLP=Int$28.90262726; CECG=Int$16.515787;

CPT =Int$8.257893502; and CBS=Int$6.193420127 (World Bank data and research,2008). Therefore, TCT 1 = (974000) × (24.77 + 28.9 +16.52 + 8.26 + 6.19) = Int$82,442,680.

Household out-of-pocket expenditures

The out-of-pocket expenses borne by patients, family members, and relatives in an nth group of countries (OOPE n) was obtained using the following formula: OOPE n = (ND n × APP n); where: ND n is the total number of people with diabetes; and APP n is the total annual spending of persons with diabetes on health care provider consultation fees, medicines, tests, transport, and other inputs. For example, in group 1 countries (ND 1 = 974000, APP1 = Int$45.7406284019997) OOPE was equal to OOPE = 974000 × 45.7406284019997 = Int $44,551,372. The average household out-of-pocket expenditures were obtained from the World Health Survey data on Mauritius for Group 1; Congo, Namibia, and Swaziland for Group 2; and Burkina Faso, Chad, Cote D'Ivoire, Comoros, Ethiopia, Ghana, Kenya, Mali, Mauritania, Malawi, Senegal, Zambia, and Zimbabwe for group 3. The monthly care expenditures were divided by the average household size of 6 members [20] to obtain expenditure per person and then multiplied by 12 to obtain the annual expenditure per person. The result was then divided by the respective country's PPP conversion rate for 2005 to obtain the international dollar equivalent (WHO Diabetic Programme, 2008).

Indirect costs

The total indirect costs (IC) of an nth group of countries were obtained using the following algorithm: IC n = (CTD n + CPD n + CPM n + CPV n); where: CTD n is the total cost of productive time lost due to diabetes related temporary disability; CPD n is the total cost of adequate time lost due to permanent disability; CPM n is the total cost of productive time lost due to diabetes-related premature mortality; and CPV n is the productivity loss due to the work time lost by relatives accompanying and visiting patients (British Medical Association, 2018).

Cost of premature diabetes-related mortality (CPM)

A total of 15692, 8636, and 88772 people died from diabetes-related causes in group 1, group 2, and group 3 countries, respectively. The distribution of those deaths across the five age brackets was obtained by multiplying the total number of diabetes deaths by the diabetes-related probabilities of death. The average age of onset and the average duration of life lived with diabetes for age brackets 0–4, 5–14, 15–44, 45–59, and 60+ years. The productive life years lost (PLYL) for 15–44, 45–59, and 60+ years age brackets were obtained by subtracting the average age of onset and average duration of life lived with diabetes from the maximum life expectancy in the African Region. The future PLYL for 0–4 and 5–14 years age brackets were calculated by subtracting the sum of the average age of onset, the average duration of life lived with diabetes, and 14 years from the maximum life expectancy in the African Region, respectively (American Diabetes Association, 1992).

The total cost of premature diabetes-related mortality (CPM) is the sum of the cost among persons aged 4 years and less, aged 5–14 years, aged 15– 44 years, 45–59 years, and aged 60+. The cost of premature diabetes related mortality among persons of a specific age group is the product of the number of deaths. The total number of productive discounted life years lost is years above 14 years of age. The gross national income per capita per year (Int$), according to American Diabetic Association (1992).

In symbolic terms, CPM for the nth age bracket can be expressed as the number of diabetes-associated deaths within its age bracket for the nth group of countries. DPYLi is the total number of discounted productive life years lost among persons of the nth age bracket, and GNIPC n is the annual gross national income per capita in PPP. The effective life years lost were discounted at 3% (Gray & Fenn, 1998).

Cost of diabetes-related permanent disability (CPD)

The total cost of productive time lost due to permanent disability (CPD n) is the sum of the effective time lost due to permanent disability among persons aged 15–44 years, 45–59 years, and 60+ years. The non-fatal illness time lost among patients below 4 years and those aged 5–14 years did not cost. The cost of productive time lost due to permanent disability among persons of various age groups was obtained by multiplying the total number of permanently disabled diabetics, discounted average duration lived with diabetes (DAD) per person, and gross national income per capita per year (PC). In symbolic terms, CPD for the nth age bracket in an nth group of countries can be expressed thus: The total cost of productive time lost due to diabetes-related temporary disability (CTD) Total productive time lost due to diabetes-related temporary disability (CTD) is the sum of the cost of effective time lost due to diabetes among persons aged 15–44 years, 45–59 years, and 60 years and over. The nonfatal illness time lost among patients aged 4 years and less and 5–14 years were not calculated. The cost of productive time lost due to diabetes-related temporary disability among persons of various age groups was obtained by multiplying the total number of temporary disabilities due to diabetes (), days of disability (DD), and daily gross national income per capita (DGNIPC n). Symbolically, the nth age bracket in an nth group of countries can be expressed thus: Cost of productive time lost by caregivers (CPV). The cost of the work time lost by accompanying/visiting relatives is a product of the number of diabetes cases (ND), the number of persons traveling to a health facility (the accompanying/visiting relatives) (VR), the number of days spent visiting a health facility per person per year (NV) and daily gross national income per capita per day (DPC).

The assumption in estimating direct and indirect costs can be found in the 'Additional file 1: Data and assumptions used in calculating indirect and direct costs of diabetes in the WHO African Region. All the cost estimates reported in chapter seven of the book are in 2005 International dollars, that is., the purchasing power parity. The indirect costs for group 2 countries amounted to Int$2,033,854,063(79.54% of total loss) worth of productive time. Out of the total indirect cost, about 88.08% was attributed to permanent disability, 1.06% to temporary disability; 9.71% to premature diabetes-associated mortality; and 1.15% to productive time lost by a family caregiver.

Average costs

An average cost per case of diabetes for groups 1, 2, and 3 countries. The averages in this table were obtained by dividing the total charges in the respective group's number of cases needing insulin, syringes, reagent strips, glucose meters, oral drugs, and hospitalization. The annual cost of insulin in the three groups of countries ranged between Int$2,064.5– $4,582.7 per diabetes case per year; the cost of syringes was Int$270.3 – $459.7 per case; the cost of reagent strips was Int$389.2 – $662.0 per case; cost of glucose meters was Int$4.9 – $8.3 per case; cost of oral drugs was Int$15.5 – $51.9 per case; cost of hospital outpatient consultations was Int$20.0 – $159.8 per case; cost of hospital admission was Int$155.0- $827.2 per case; cost of diabetes test Int$84.6 – $188.1 per case; health care cost borne by households as US$45.7– $88.3percase; cost of productive time lost was Int$10,168.9– $116,215.1 per permanently disabled case; cost of adequate time lost was Int$10.6 –$121.7 per temporarily disabled case, and cost of proper time lost was Int$10.7 – $121.8 per caregiver. The cost of productive time lost per premature death ranged between Int$ 5,565.0 in Group 3 and $63,599.6 in Group 1 countries.

The average cost per person with diabetes in groups 1, 2, and 3. These averages were obtained by dividing the itemized total costs in Tables 2 by 974000, 536000, and 5510000 diabetes cases in groups 1, 2, and 3, respectively. The annual cost of insulin was Int$309.7 – $687.4 per diabetes patient; the cost of syringes was Int$40.5 – $69.0 per diabetes patient. The cost of reagent strips was Int$58.4 – $99.3 per diabetes patient; the cost of glucose meters was Int$0.7 – $ 1.2 per diabetes patient. The cost of oral drugs was Int$13.2 – $44.1 per diabetes patient; the cost of hospital outpatient consultations was Int$20.0 – $159.8 per diabetes patient; the cost of hospital admission was Int$23.3-$141.0 per diabetes patient; the cost of diabetes test Int$84.6 – $188.1 per diabetes patient. Health care cost borne by households was Int$45.7 – $88.3 per diabetes patient; cost of productive time lost was Int$813.5 – $9297.2 per diabetes patient; cost of adequate time lost was Int$9.8 – $111.9 per diabetes patient; and cost of proper time lost was Int$89.7 – $1024.7 per diabetes patient. The cost of productive time lost due to premature death was Int$2144.3 – $11431.6 per diabetes patient.

Average cost per person with diabetes (Int$) in 2005

The 7.02 million cases of diabetes recorded by countries of the African Region in 2000 resulted in a total economic loss of Int $25.51 billion, that is, $3633 per patient with diabetes. About 43.65%, 10.03%, and 46.32% of that loss were incurred by groups 1, 2, and 3 countries, respectively. Group 1 has only six countries that control a relatively substantial amount of wealth, which largely accounts for the high economic burden of diabetes. There were 33 countries with the lowest GNI per capita. It bore 78% of the total burden of diabetes in the Region and the highest economic burden of diabetes. The total annual costs associated with diabetes in

Latin America and the Caribbean were estimated at US$65.216 billion.

The total indirect cost was about Int$8.1 billion, 32% in the Region, that is 1,154.15 per diabetes patient. The direct price in corroding treating diabetes was Int$ 853.2 million in Group 1, Int$ 523.3 million in Group 2, and Int$ 6.7 billion in Group 3. The main driver of direct cost across the three groups was the total number of people needing insulin. On the other hand, the indirect cost of diabetes amounted to Int$10.3 billion in Group 1, Int$2.03 billion in Group 2, and Int$5.09 billion in Group 3. Permanent disability accounted for 81.33%, 70.06%, and 37.94% of the total indirect costs in groups 1, 2, and 3, respectively. Intuitively, this is understandable, given the chronic nature of diabetes disease. This finding is closely similar to that of Barceló et al. [4], which found that indirect costs accounted for 82% of the total charges in Latin America and the Caribbean.

The accuracy of these estimates hinges on the plausibility of the assumptions contained in the 'Additional file 1: Data and assumptions used in estimating indirect and direct costs of diabetes in the WHO African Region, and their interpretation should be tempered with the limitations highlighted below. The reader should keep in mind that the purpose of the total cost of illness studies, such as the one reported in this paper, is not to guide policy decisions but to raise awareness among policymakers and the public about the negative economic impact of diabetes. In the above calculation of the cost of diabetes, there was total disregard for complications in the price of the burden associated with diabetes. Various complications such as retinopathy, cardiovascular diseases, nephropathy, and peripheral vascular disease are associated with diabetes—most of the deaths related to diabetes result from those complications. However, it was impossible to directly estimate their cost due to a lack of information on such difficulties for the African Region. Therefore, it is likely that we will have underestimated the economic burden of diabetes mellitus in African countries by disregarding such complications.

The assumption is that those who suffer from diabetes, disability, and mortality would have future earnings. In this book, it is assumed that all those who are temporarily or permanently disabled by diabetes or die from causes associated with diabetes would have future earnings. Based on this assumption, it can be contested in African countries where the formal sectors are small. Thus the proportion of people in formal employment is small. In situations where The unemployment rate is high, the marginal labor productivity might be less than the average. In this case, the use of Gross National Income (GNI) per capita may likely overestimate the economic burden of diabetes in Africa.

Use of the human capital approach

It is an approach that values health benefits in terms of the present value of future lost output as measured commonly by earnings and other labor costs. This approach values health benefits in terms of production gained due to a decrease in mortality in terms of loss of productive years, morbidity resulting in loss of working time, and debility leading to loss of productive capacity at work. Therefore, the human capital approach assumes that the objective function society is trying to maximize through improved health is Gross National Income. And wages in the African Region are a good indicator of productivity. The approach has been criticized for not being consistent with the primary rationale of the economic calculus used in cost-benefit analysis. The potential Pareto optimality; and the fact that people value prevention of premature death, morbidity, and incapacity per se rather than their concern to preserve productive resources and maintain future levels of GNP.

Omission of intangible example, many African communities may be opposed to getting married in families with a history of diabetes, which may have enormous psychological costs on the families concerned. Unfortunately, since most of the data used in this study were obtained from secondary sources, it was not possible to conduct a household survey that would have made it possible to estimates the intangible costs using a contingent willingness-to-pay approach.

Use of per capita GNI value-productive time lost.

This book treated the loss in the Gross National Income (GNI) and not the total economic cost of disability and premature mortality associated with diabetes. The social value of women's contribution to African societies is more significant than that captured in GNI calculations. This is because the International Labour Organization's (ILO) definition of labor force includes the employed, such as the armed forces, the unemployed, and the first-time job-seekers, but excludes full-time homemakers and other unpaid caregivers and workers in the informal sector. Most of the women in Africa are full-time homemakers and casual sector workers. Therefore, their invaluable contribution to society is excluded from GNI calculations.

Despite data limitations, the estimates reported here show that diabetes imposes a substantive economic burden on countries of the African Region. That heavy burden underscores the urgent need for increased investments to fully implement the WHO Regional Committee for Africa, World Health Assembly, and United Nations General Assembly resolutions on preventing and controlling diabetes.

In addition, given the high degree of ignorance about the magnitude of the epidemiological and economic burdens of diabetes mellitus in the WHO African Region, there is an urgent need for further research to determine: the national-level epidemiological burden of diabetes, measured in terms of its prevalence, incidence, mortality, and, probably, disability-adjusted life years lost; national-level economic burden of diabetes, broken down by differences.

Prevalence Of Neonatal Diabetes Mellitus

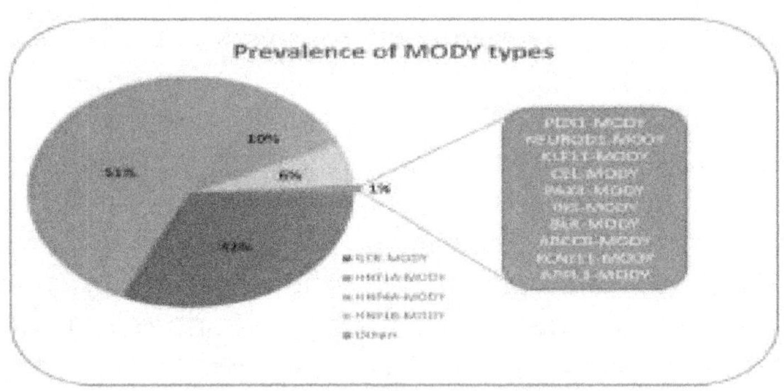

Without existing data, the book intends to treat the incidence, prevalence, and genetic determinants of neonatal Diabetes mellitus (NDM) with an expected contribution to disease characterization.

It includes cross-sectional, cohort, or case-control studies that reported NDM's incidence, prevalence, and genetic determinants without geographical limitations. Clinical heterogeneity was adopted to examine the design and setting (including geographic region), the procedure used for genetic testing, the calculation of incidence or prevalence, and outcomes in each study to determine the majority of neonatal diabetes in selected study areas.

Systematic review and meta-analysis are expected to draw a clear picture of phenotypic and genotypic presentations of NDM to understand the condition better and adequately address the challenges concerning its management. Neonatal Diabetes mellitus (NDM) is a severe and monogenic form of Diabetes mellitus (DM), characterized by the onset of insulin-requiring hyperglycemia within the first months of life. NDM may be transient or permanent. Transient NDM presents soon after birth and undergoes spontaneous remission during infancy. It may relapse to a permanent form of DM in childhood or adolescence, making it a temporary state of neonatal Diabetes mellitus. Permanent NDM, which accounts for 40–50% of cases of NDM, occurs during the first six months of life and does not go into remission, with patients often presenting the following symptoms:

- Vomiting
- Dehydration
- Poor feeding
- Hyperglycemia
- Ketosis

Neonatal Diabetes mellitus (NDM) has been estimated to occur in out of 20,000 to 500,000 live births, but no precise estimate is specific. The etiology of NDM can be attributed to the non-existing or disturbed development of the pancreas, reduced pancreatic β cell mass, disturbed β cell function, or early Islet of Langerhans of liver destruction.

There is strong evidence that a genetic diagnosis of NDM improves the treatment. For instance, neonates suffering from NDM caused by a potassium channel gene mutation are susceptible to sulphonylurea treatment. Therefore, replacing insulin with oral agents can improve their clinical management. Traditional genetic testing for NDM will require accurate clinical information about the patient's phenotype to allow the selection of a small number of genes to test. However, selecting genes to be sequenced will also require a predictive list based on what is usually already registered. No existing data has yet compiled the phenotypic and genotypic presentations of both forms of NDM and the factors determining their occurrence. It is believed that a study addressing this issue is highly needed. It will generate significant clinical impact in terms of a better characterization of the disease subtypes followed by improvement in NDM management. It is essential to understand the following in the management of neonatal diabetes:

- The incidence of NDM
- The prevalence of NDM

- The genetic and epigenetic determinants of NDM

Peer-reviewed original reports of observational studies (cross-sectional, cohort, or case-control studies) on the incidence, prevalence, genetic, and epigenetic determinants of NDM were systematically identified and appraised by researchers. These must have been conducted on human subjects without any geographical limitation. Neonatal Diabetes mellitus incidence is influenced by geographical locations and the genetic makeup of the neonatal. It has been found through various studies that where children are born may influence the prevalence of NDM in such children. Where substantial heterogeneity will be detected in the study of neonatal diabetes, a subgroup analysis will be performed using the following grouping variables: geographical region, assessment strategy, a subtype of NDM, age at diagnosis, and study methodological quality. The findings are summarized in a narrative if the included studies differ significantly in design, settings, and outcome measures. This systematic review and meta-analysis are expected to draw a clear picture of phenotypic and genotypic presentations of NDM to understand the condition better and adequately address challenges concerning its management. This review does not require ethical approval since it is based on published studies and not individual participant data. Its results will be published in a peer-reviewed journal and shared at relevant scientific conferences.

There is genetically induced neonatal diabetes. There have been different assertions in the past 100 years about the genetic causes of diabetes in newborns, infants, adolescents, and adults. Generally, the disease is known to be chronic at a particular stage of its morbidity. Recent research findings have associated Diabetes mellitus with specific genotypes. Diabetes is a lifelong chronic disease. During the past 100 years, its diagnosis has been based on measurements of raised blood glucose concentrations. In the 1960s, diabetes was classified based on age and need for insulin treatment (juvenile or maturity-onset; insulin or non-insulin-requiring diabetes). As a result of the general belief that diabetes is an inherited disease, much hope was placed on identifying genetic markers that would help diagnose diabetic subgroups. However, scientists in the 1970s noted that type 1 diabetes was strongly associated with the HLA locus on chromosome 6, which is a determination of HLA genotypes but failed to add substantial diagnostic value because of their high Prevalence.

The discovery of autoantibodies to different islet antigens in the 1980s added discriminatory solid power to the autoimmune type 1 diabetes diagnosis. This new knowledge was later applied to adults' late-onset autoimmune forms of diabetes. The first real genetic breakthroughs in diabetes classification came with the discovery that mutations in the genes encoding glucokinase, HNF1A, and HNF4A were associated with different forms of maturity-onset diabetes of the young.

While maturity-onset diabetes of the young can show varying prevalence and severity, neonatal diabetes, which is rare(1:100000 births), a severe form of diabetes, is diagnosed in infants younger than 6 months. A group in Exeter in the United Kingdom pioneered the genetic dissection of neonatal diabetes and noted that one form could be linked to mutations in the KCNJ11 gene in encoding the Kir6.2 subunit of the ATP-dependent potassium channel in pancreatic cells. It could be treated with sulphonylureas, the study further stated. During the past 20 years, more than 20 genes have been identified as causing neonatal diabetes.

In many of these monogenic diseases, a causal diagnosis has had an essential effect on the choice of treatment and disease outcome. In one striking case, after identifying a mutation in the KCNJ11 gene in a malnourished child with neonatal diabetes and switching from insulin to large doses of sulphonylurea, the child's diabetes could not be well controlled. Still, development, walking, and talking became possible. Kir6.2 is also expressed in the brain, and this combination of diabetes, developmental brain defects, and sometimes epilepsy has been called developmental delay-epilepsy-neonatal diabetes. There is clear evidence of the existence of a genetic diagnosis improving treatment.

However, in patients diagnosed with maturity-onset diabetes of the young, those with mutations in the glucokinase gene do not need any treatment. Because the transformation only modestly raises the threshold for the phosphorylating capacity of the enzyme. Therefore, a slight increase in glucose can fully overcome this defect.

However, maturity-onset diabetes of the young caused by glucokinase mutations is not a disease but a compensated metabolic disorder.

A patient received a diagnosis of diabetes as a child, but, after many years and about 19000 insulin injections, received a precise genetic diagnosis that a mutation in the glucokinase gene caused her diabetes. Now, she needs no treatment. The Exeter group has not only pioneered research in this field but also removed barriers by providing free genetic tests to patients from many different countries. Research grants fund it.

In the early days of the study in 2000, genetic testing was expensive and time-consuming. Therefore, the scientists used Sanger sequencing of selected genes based on previous clinical information. The addition of targeted next-generation sequencing to Sanger sequencing in 2012 reduced the cost and time required and broadened the range of variants that could be tested without clinical data. This change culminated in identifying a genetic diagnosis in 82% (840/1020) of tested patients.

Consequently, most patients are now referred within weeks of being diagnosed with diabetes, physicians can achieve a nearly genetic diagnosis and predict the development of associated clinical features. De Franco and colleagues have documented the clinical benefit of early diagnosis and treatment in specific subgroups of patients with neonatal diabetes. This approach still requires a prediction of the genes to sequence, which is reasonable in neonatal diabetes (i.e., with an apparent phenotype of diagnosis of diabetes <6 months of age), but not all cases of monogenic diabetes are this clear-cut. The next step in less clear clinical situations will be whole-genome sequencing without any assumptions about what genes might be involved. Although cost is a restriction in this situation, this whole-genome sequencing approach can already work for rare recessive mutations. We recently identified three recessive mutations in BBZ10 causing the Bardet-Biedl syndrome in an analysis of next-generation sequence data from Finland.

The three adult carriers had not been diagnosed with the syndrome, even though clinical features meant that Bardet-Biedl syndrome could not be excluded. However, many challenges must be overcome before whole genome sequencing becomes part of routine clinical work-up in different specialties. Hopefully, the UK Government's 100000 Genome Project and the US$215 million promised by former President Obama to create a Precision Medicine Initiative in the USA to provide impetus towards this goal. Such projects should lead to more precise diagnoses informing treatment in different genetically-determined diseases and increase the number of affected individuals who will benefit from diagnosis and treatment. Pancreatic beta cells express two auto-antigenic forms of glutamic acid decarboxylase, a 65-kDa hydrophilic form, and a 64-kDa amphiphilic form; both are membrane-bound and soluble. Antibodies to glutamic acid decarboxylase reveal latent autoimmune Diabetes mellitus Mutations in the hepatocyte nuclear factor-1α gene in the onset of diabetes.

The effect of early, comprehensive genomic testing on clinical care in neonatal diabetes: an international cohort study neonatal Diabetes (ND) Mellitus is a rare genetic disease (1 in 90,000 live births). It is defined by the presence of severe hyperglycemia associated with insufficient or no circulating insulin, occurring mainly before 6 months of age and rarely between 6 months and 1 year. Such hyperglycemia requires either transient treatment with insulin in about half of the cases or permanent insulin treatment. The disease is explained by two influential groups of mechanisms: malformation of the pancreas with altered insulin-secreting cells development/survival or abnormal function of the existing pancreatic β cell. The most frequent genetic causes of neonatal diabetes mellitus with abnormal β cell function are abnormalities of the 6q24 locus and mutations of the ABCC8orKCNJ11 genes coding for the potassium channel in the pancreatic β cell. Other genes are associated with pancreas malformation, insufficient β cell development, or destruction of β cells.

Clinically, compared to patients with an ABCC8 or KCNJ11 mutation, patients with a 6q24 abnormality have lower birth weight and height, are younger at diagnosis and remission, and have higher malformation frequency. Patients with an ABCC8 or KCNJ11 mutation have neurological and neuropsychological disorders in all those tested carefully. Up to 86% of patients who go into remission have recurrent diabetes when they reach puberty, with no difference due to their genetic origin. All these results reinforce the importance of prolonged follow-up by a multidisciplinary pediatric team, and later doctors specializing in adult medicine.90% of the patients with an ABCC8orKCNJ11 mutation and those with 6q24 anomalies are amenable to a successful switch from insulin injection to oral sulfonylureas.

Diabetes mellitus in very young children or neonatal diabetes is a rare genetic disease (minimal incidence: 1 in 90,000 live births) with variations within different ethnic groups. It is defined by the presence of severe hyperglycemia requiring treatment and occurs between the neonatal period and infancy. It appears mainly months of age (155/173 probands in our published cohort) and rarely between 6 months and 1 year (18/173). In the Finnish population, for example, after 6 months of age, patients with diabetes had high HLA risk genotypes and islet autoantibodies, reflecting the autoimmune character of diabetes. This hyperglycemia is associated with insufficient or no circulating insulin. Two clinical forms have been distinguished based on the duration of the treatment: a so-called "transient form" and a permanent form.

Two influential groups of mechanisms explain the disease: malformation of the pancreas or abnormal function of the pancreatic β cell that secretes insulin by poor insulin cell mass development or malfunction of a cell component or by the destruction of the β cell. Genetic causes of monogenic neonatal diabetes based on physiopathological mechanisms [excluding 6q24 locus abnormalities. **Mechanism of insulin secretion in response to glucose and glibenclamide.**

Abnormal β Cell Function

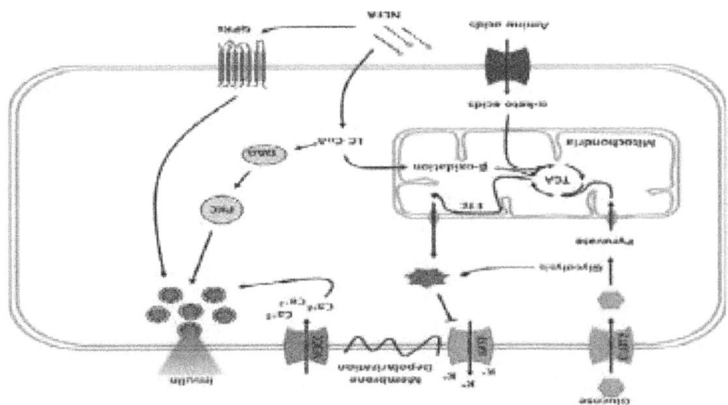

The most frequent genetic causes of neonatal diabetes with normal pancreas morphology are abnormalities of the 6q24 locus and mutations of the genes coding for the ATP-dependent potassium channel. The first genetic causes identified were abnormalities of the 6q24 locus, which include paternal uniparental disomy of 6q24 (pUPD6), partial duplication of paternal 6q24, and relaxation of the maternal 6q24 imprinted locus. This locus contains a CpG island, presenting differential methylation depending on the parental origin (non-methylation on the paternal allele, methylation on the maternal allele).

To date, methylation abnormality has not been found in the parents of affected children. Methylation is used to down-regulate gene transcription of the methylated allele. All these abnormalities lead to the over-expression of imprinted genes located in 6q24, such as PLAGL1/ZAC (pleiomorphic adenoma gene-like 1) and HYMAI (Hydatidi form mole-associated and imprinted transcript), which are the most "likely" candidate genes.

PLAGL-1 codes for a transcription factor involved in the regulation of stopping the cell cycle and apoptosis and in the induction of the receptor 1 gene for human pituitary adenylate cyclase-activating polypeptide (PACAP1, which is a potent stimulant of insulin secretion).

The function of the HYMAI gene is unknown. The mechanism responsible for diabetes could be linked to a developmental defect in the β cells. Still, the fact that remission of diabetes occurs means that an abnormality in β cell function cannot be ruled out. The 6q24 abnormalities are associated with "transient" neonatal diabetes.

The ZFP57 gene (MIM *612192) is involved in maintaining methylation of the DNA during the very early stages of embryogenesis. It is localized at 6p22.1. Homozygous mutations leading to a lack of protein or nonfunctional protein are associated with widespread DNA hypomethylation, including hypo methylation of the 6q24 locus.

However, some patients have a 6q24 methylation abnormality, not due to mutations of this gene. The ATP-dependent potassium channel (KATP channel) plays a central role in stimulating insulin secretion by the pancreatic β cell in response to glucose. At low blood sugar levels (e.g., fasting), the KATP channels are open (activated), and their activity maintains a hyperpolarized resting membrane potential (around −70 mV). A rise in blood sugar level (e.g., post-prandial) causes the increased passage of glucose into the β cell. Glucose enters the glycolysis pathway, which increases the intracellular ATP concentration.

It causes the KATP channels to close (inhibition), which leads to intracellular potassium accumulation that causes membrane depolarization. This depolarization activates the 2+voltage-dependent calcium channels, leading to ions entering the β cell, then exocytosis of the secretion vesicles and insulin release into the bloodstream. The KATP channel is an octamer formed from two types of subunits: the Kir6.2 subunits form the channel selective for the incoming corrective potassium enclosed in SUR1 ion-channel regulator subunits. They are coded by the KCNJ11 and ABCC8 genes, respectively. Activating mutations in one of these two genes are responsible for neonatal diabetes with normal pancreas morphology. They result in the KATP channel remaining permanently open so that it no longer controls membrane potential in response to glucose and therefore blocks the event cascade that leads to insulin release.

By frequency, the third cause of neonatal diabetes is mutations of the insulin gene (INS). The majority are heterozygous mutations affecting the structure of PR proinsulin; these are transmitted in an autosomal dominant manner. The abnormal proinsulin undergoes degradation in the endoplasmic reticulum, leading to severe endoplasmic reticulum (ER) stress and β cell death. This process has been described in mouse models and man. Recent evidence suggests that INS mutations do not necessarily lead to beta-cell death, but relatively chronic ER stress interferes with beta-cell growth and development.

Some mutations alter the expression of the protein. They are transmitted in a recessive manner in the majority of cases in consanguineous families. These mutations affect the insulin promoter directly or by a mutation in the factor that enhances its activity.

Mutations of the Glucokinase Gene

Glucokinase is responsible for the first step of glucose metabolism in the β cell. It acts as a "sensor" of blood glucose, making it possible to control the quantity of insulin secreted. Nonsense mutations of the glucokinase gene cause MODY 2 (Maturity onset diabetes in the youth type 2), which usually presents as moderate hyperglycemia. Transmission is heterozygous. In the homozygous state, these nonsense mutations cause neonatal diabetes by complete deficiency of glucokinase-mediated glycolysis. It is not a frequent cause of neonatal diabetes. However, an assay of the fasting blood glucose concentration is required from both parents, mainly if there is a history of gestational diabetes. The discovery of discreet glucose intolerance in both parents should therefore lead to a search for glucokinase gene mutations.

Abnormal Pancreas Morphology

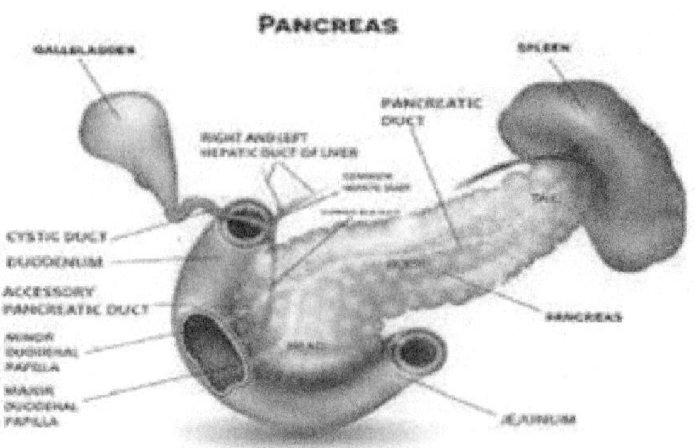

Several genes are linked to neonatal diabetes with abnormal pancreas morphology, and a detailed description is beyond the scope of this chapter. These genes are involved in the development of the pancreas at various stages in early morphogenesis. These neonatal diabetes cases may be associated with a deficiency of the exocrine pancreas based on the severity of pancreatic damage or other congenital malformations. Mutation of the RFX-6 gene deserves specific comment. The RFX-6 transcription factor is involved in the differentiation of beta-cells in the pancreas during embryonic development. It is also expressed in mature cells, where it has a role in regulating insulin transcription and secretion. It controls the expression and activation of calcium channels, and its inactivation alters insulin secretion in response to glucose. Patients display developmental abnormalities of the pancreas and the digestive tract. The mechanism is linked to a developmental and functional disorder of the endocrine pancreas. Transmission is autosomal recessive.

Autoimmune Neonatal Diabetes Mellitus

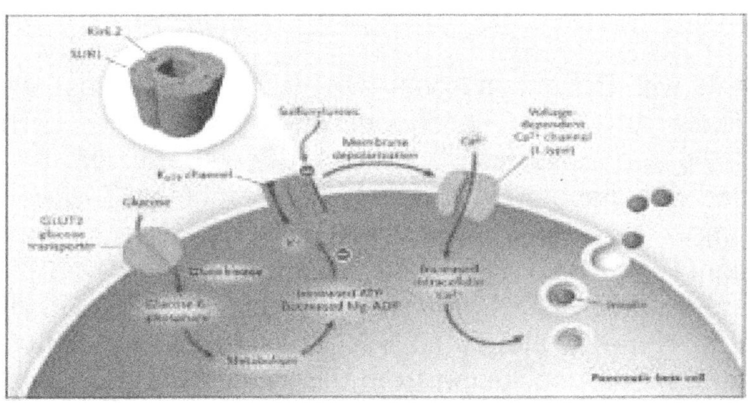

Most patients with diabetes between 6 and 12 months of age will have the "typical" type 1 diabetes mellitus seen in older children with positive autoantibodies against the beta cell. Autoimmune diabetes is rare before 6 months of age and is most often linked to specific causes. Mutations of the FOXP3 gene may be responsible for entero-pathy, immune dysregulation, and polyendocrinopathy. It is a cause of neonatal diabetes associated with early autoimmunity directed against the beta cells of the pancreas. This diagnosis should be considered in male infants presenting diabetes related to immune deficiency and severe infections. Immuno-suppressant treatment (sirolimus, corticosteroids) can be considered, but a bone marrow transplant must be regarded as soon as the child's clinical condition allows. Insulin treatment will be combined with specialized nutritional management (parenteral ± enteral nutrition) before and after the transplant. It should be noted that correcting immune deficiencies will not eliminate diabetes.

The relationship between Down Syndrome and Neonatal Diabetes Mellitus

Patients with Down syndrome (DS) resulting from trisomy 21 are more likely to have childhood diabetes mellitus. Professor Hattersley's group found 13 infants affected by DS who were diagnosed with diabetes before the age of 6 months. Trisomy 21 was seven times more likely in their PNDM cohort than in the general population(13of 1,522 = 85 of 10,000 observed vs. 12.6 of 10,000 expected). Known PNDM genes explain 82.9% of non-DS PNDM in their work. None of the 13 DS-PNDM patients had a mutation in those genes. The conclusion from this work is that trisomy 21 is a cause of autoimmune PNDM that is not HLA associated. Other modifications, such as the activating STAT3 mutations have been described which cause neonatal diabetes associated with beta cell autoimmunity.

Clinical Explanation

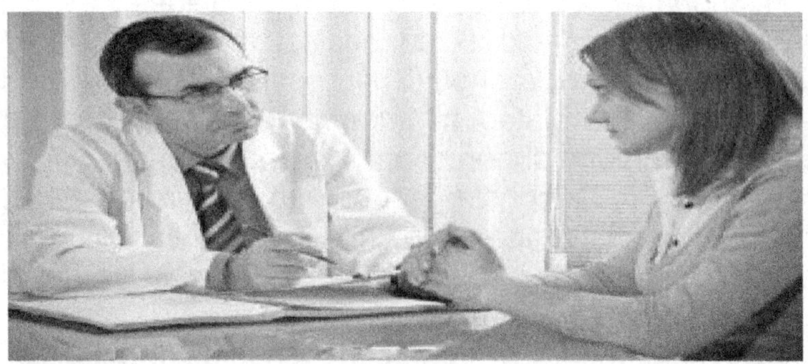

There are two clinical forms of neonatal diabetes based on the duration of insulin dependency. In short, treatment may be stopped anytime from the first weeks of life to 5 years of age. In permanent structures, life-long therapy is necessary. Distinct molecular mechanisms do not always underpin the clinical difference between transient and permanent neonatal diabetes. Abnormalities of the 6q24 locus are exclusively linked to transient neonatal diabetes. However, mutations of the ABCC8, KCNJ11, and INS genes are linked to both permanent and temporary forms. Other genetic causes are associated with permanent neonatal diabetes.

Neonatal diabetes is usually diagnosed before 6 months of age. However, the age of diagnosis varies depending on genetic causes: diabetes due to a 6q24 locus abnormality appears before the age of 1 month in 93% of cases and before the period of 3 months in 100% of cases. InABCC8andKCNJ11gene mutations, it appears before 1 month in 30% of cases and between 1 and 6 months in 66% of cases. At birth, patients have a birth weight below the 10th percentile in 62% of cases, highlighting the crucial role of insulin secretion in fetal growth. This intrauterine growth retardation is found in all genetic groups, with a greater proportion in patients with a 6q24 abnormality than those carrying an ABCC8orKCNJ11 mutation (92 vs. 48%,$p< 0.001$). Half of the patients with a detectable pancreas by ultrasound experience remission from diabetes in our cohort. It occurs at the age of about 4 months. There is a difference depending on the genetic cause. Patients with a 6q24 locus abnormality are in remission before the age of 1 year in 97% of cases (median age 14 weeks), while remission may go as far as the age of 5 years in patients with an ABCC8orKCNJ11 mutation (median age 39 weeks). Patients with a rare recessive mutation of the INS gene have remission at a median age of 12 weeks, while most of the INS gene mutations are dominant and never go into remission. Diabetes frequent relapses (in up to 86% of cases) at the onset of puberty, probably due to the insulin resistance of puberty. There is no difference between the genetic groups. Depending on the genetic cause, patients with neonatal diabetes may have other clinical signs associated with diabetes.

In neonatal diabetes with normal pancreas morphology, there are associated neurological disorders and developmental defects. Approximately 25% of patients with a mutation of the ABCC8orKCNJ11 genes have neurological diseases ranging from psychomotor disorders to delayed cognitive development associated with severe epilepsy (DEND syndrome: Developmental delay, Epilepsy, and Neonatal Diabetes). In addition, we have shown when patients undergo detailed neuro psychomotor and neuropsychological tests, an attention deficit or language disorder extending as far as dyslexia is found in 100% of cases. Patients with a 6q24 locus abnormality may have developmental defects (macroglossia, umbilical hernia, cardiac malformations, renal and urinary malformations, non-autoimmune anemia, and hypothyroidism with gland in situ) and neurological disorders.

In neonatal diabetes with abnormal pancreas morphology or β cell destruction, the associated malformations depend on the genetic causes and are often grouped into defined syndromes.

Is Diabetes Becoming An Epidemic?

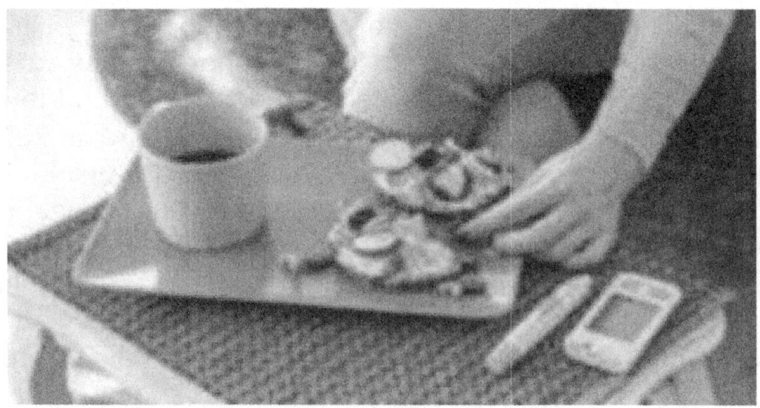

Type 2 Diabetes appears to be assuming an epidemic proportion in developed and developing countries. It occurs due to the body's resistance to insulin, which builds up sugar in the blood. Type 2 diabetes is commonly associated with lifestyles. There are other kinds of type 2 diabetes which for the avoidance of ambiguity are given nomenclature based on who and how they exhibit their symptoms on the patients. Pre-diabetes is a type 2 Diabetes

mellitus that occurs when the blood sugar level rises above average but not to the fatality level or poses a danger to the individual. Another one worth mentioning is gestational diabetes which occurs in some pregnant women. It is called gestational diabetes because it occurs within the nine months gestation period of a pregnant woman. It is associated with an insulin-blocking hormone that is produced by the placenta. That is why it does not occur in early pregnancy until about three months after the pregnancy when the fetus must have developed a placenta. When gestational diabetes occurs in conjunction with gestational hypertension in a pregnant woman, the risk of developing clamps is very high. The excellent news about gestational diabetes is that it goes with delivery. As soon as the pregnant woman puts to bed, the blood sugar level becomes normal. It is advisable for the pregnant woman who has gestational diabetes to attend an antenatal clinic where the Community Health Nurse and gynecologist will offer professional care to manage the condition until the pregnant woman gives birth. Diabetes insipidus is another type of type 2 diabetes which is a condition in which the kidney removes a copious amount of fluid from the body. Unlike Diabetes mellitus, there is no sugar in the urine of the person suffering from this Diabetes insipidus. Both diabetic conditions have their unique symptoms, causes, and control.

My Carbohydrate Guide

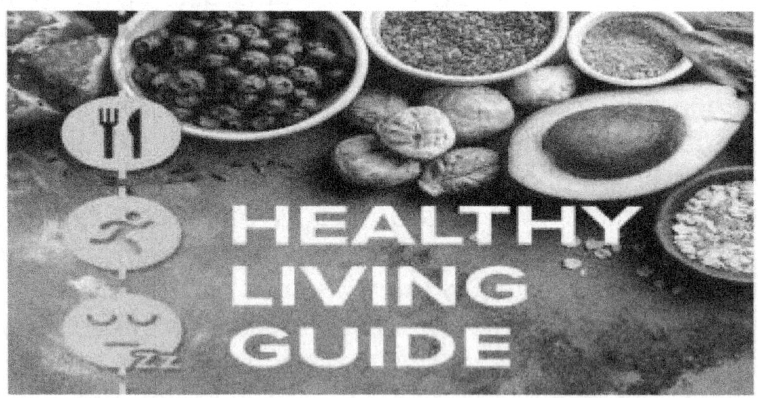

Diabetes Care and Education (DCE), an Academy of Nutrition and Dietetics dietetic practice group promotes quality diabetes care and education. DCE comprises Academy of Nutrition and Dietetics members who are experts in medical nutrition therapy and diabetes care. Their expertise is widely acknowledged in the diabetes community. We are excited to be able to work with this group of professionals on the development of My Carbohydrate Guide. I hope you find it to be a helpful resource.

What Are Carbohydrates

Carbohydrates (also called carbs) are one of three cue nutrients or building blocks that comprise all foods. Protein and fat are the other two building blocks. To be healthy and strong, your body requires all three. Many foods restrain a combination of carbohydrates, protein, and fat. Blood sugar also called blood glucose, is formed from the carbohydrates we consume and is used as an energy source by the cells.

Regarding diabetes, carbs get the most attention because they raise blood sugar levels when your body digests. Many carbohydrate-containing foods are nutritious. They taste fine and provide calories and energy to fuel your body, as well as crucial vitamins, minerals, and fiber your body needs.

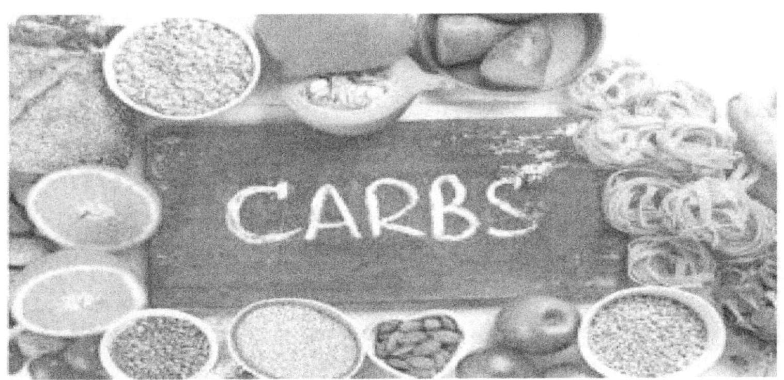

What Foods Contain Carbs?

- Bread, cereals, and grains
- Crackers and snacks
- Dried beans, peas, and lentils
- Fruits
- Milk and yogurt
- No starchy vegetables
- Starchy vegetables
- Sweets, desserts, and regular soda

Why Do You Need to Know About Carbohydrates- Rich Foods If You Have Diabetes?

When you consume carbohydrates, your body breaks them down, causing your blood sugar levels to rise. Different carbohydrate amounts have other effects on blood sugar levels. A high-carbohydrate meal (such as a plate of pasta and a breadstick) will raise blood sugar levels more than a low-carbohydrate meal (such as grilled chicken breast, salad, and broccoli). Insulin is a hormone that is produced by the pancreas. The body uses insulin to transport glucose from the bloodstream into cells, which is used for vitality. If you possess type 2 diabetes, your body can have difficulty utilizing your insulin, or your pancreas may produce insufficient insulin. Your pancreas doesn't produce insulin if you have type 1 diabetes. Eating the right amount of carbohydrates at each meal and taking diabetes medications, including insulin, if necessary, may help keep your blood sugar levels closer to target.

How Many Carbohydrates Should You Consume?

Your registered specialist can advise you on how many carbs you require. The amount is determined by age, weight, activity level, and diabetes medications if any are worn. You can learn how "counting carbs" at each meal (and snacks, if necessary) can help you stay within your blood sugar target range. Consult your registered dietitian or healthcare provider to determine the appropriate number of carbs for you. Carbohydrates are a crucial component of a healthy diet. It's critical to watch your portion sizes and get most of your carbs from fruits, vegetables, whole grains, low-fat milk, and yogurt.

Sample meal with four carbs options:

- 1 whole wheat bread slice (1 carb choice)
- ½ cup mashed potatoes (1 carbohydrate option)
- ½ cup mashed potatoes (1 carbohydrate option)
- 1-quart skim milk (1 carb choice)

- To round out the meal, include the following foods, which will primarily provide nutrients other than carbs:
- 3 oz. of chicken (0 carb choices)
- 1 salad (green) (0 carb choices)
- 1–2 tablespoons dressing (0 carb choices)

How Much Do You Eat?

A part is the quantity of food you consume. It may differ from the serving size listed on the Nutrition Facts label of a food. Food label serving sizes are standardized to make it easier to compare similar foods. They come in standard sizes, such as cups or pieces. The serving size decides the number of calories, carbs, and other nutrients listed on the food label.

Take note of the serving size and the number of servings in the food package. "How many servings am I eating?" Ask yourself. You can eat 12 servings, 1 serving, or more of whatever you want. You can be eating more carbohydrates than you realize. As a result, carefully examine the Nutrition Facts label to estimate the number of carbs you get from food.

Food portion sizes are increasing, making it easy to lose sight of what constitutes a standard serving size. Furthermore, the larger the portion offered, the more people consume! Portion sizes can be big than what a person requires at one time, so to help manage your diabetes, be aware of the measures and carb content of foods and beverages.

A Handy Guide to Portion Sizes

Use this quick guide to estimate portion sizes and carbs to stay on track with your portions. Practice can assist you in learning portion sizes that provide the number of carbs you require to keep your blood sugar levels stable. Your palm, excluding your fingers and thumb, is approximately 3 ounces of cooked and boneless meat. For foods like ice cream or cooked cereal, a fist equals about 1 cup or 30 grams of carbs. 1 tablespoon or 1 serving of orderly salad dressing, low-fat mayonnaise, or low-fat margarine equals your thumb. Your thumb tip is 1 teaspoon or one serving of margarine, mayonnaise, or other fats such as oils.

These portion estimates are based on the size of a woman's hand. Hand sizes differ. Portion estimates will vary depending on the size of the hand used. Measuring or weighing foods is the most precise way to determine portion size.

What Is Healthy Eating?

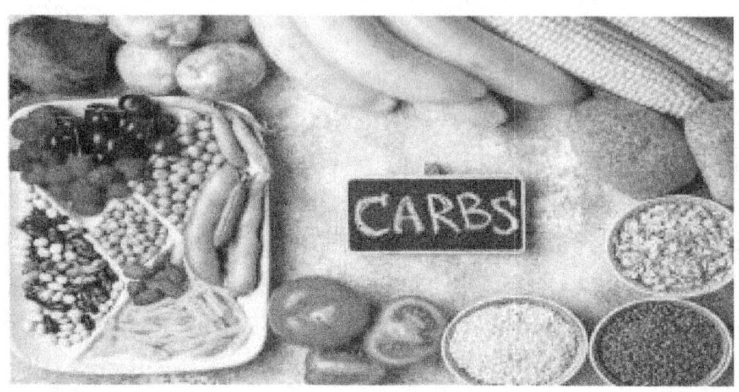

Healthy eating is defined as eating only what your body requires—not too much or too little of one type of food or beverage. Pick fruits, vegetables, whole grains, and low-fat or non-fat dairy products for most of your carbs. In your meal planning, choose lower-fat meats and limit fats, oils, sweets, and alcohol. When you have diabetes, you can benefit from eating lower-fat, higher-fiber foods, and just enough calories to keep healthy. Eating fruits and vegetables of all colors also provide essential vitamins and minerals. Most foods can be included in a healthy meal plan. Everything is dependent on the following:

How much
How frequently
What else do you intend to eat

Is it too little or too much?

People frequently consume excessive amounts of these:
Total fat, saturated fat, trans fat, cholesterol, and sodium are all factors to consider (salt). Some people can't get enough of these: Iron, calcium, fiber, vitamins A, C, and D. Eating 2 to 3 cups of vegetables and 112 to 2 cups of fruit daily to get enough vitamins, minerals, and fiber. Eating three servings of fat-free or low-fat dairy foods daily to get enough calcium.

Association of parameters with diabetic retinopathy

Significant demographical parameters, clinical conditions, and laboratory tests has been studied in the multivariate analyses for the prediction of association with retinopathy and age, male sex, hypertension, duration of Diabetes mellitus, presence of diabetic neuropathy, presence of diabetic nephropathy, presence of diabetic foot ulcer, foot amputation, fasting blood glucose, serum total cholesterol, serum triglyceride and HbA1care associated with diabetic retinopathy.

The study conducted on diabetic retinopathy shows that it is the most frequent ocular fundus disease. Diabetic Mellitus patients with retinopathy have elevated blood chemistry, hypertension, nephropathy, neuropathy, and/or a foot ulcer as well as a long duration of diabetes. The results of the study are consistent with a study on a Chinese community. Poor vision and blindness are severe public health problems in China due to diabetic neuropathy that has resulted in retinopathy. Monitoring of blood parameters and early screening of ocular fundus diseases are required in a long duration of diabetes mellitus to prevent damage to the eyes.

The study reported age, male sex, hypertension, duration of diabetes, diabetic neuropathy, diabetic nephropathy, presence of diabetic foot ulcer, and foot amputation as independent risk factors for diabetic retinopathy. The results of the study are consistent with multi-hospital-based cross-sectional studies of the Chinese community. Aging and other comorbidities have a significant association with the prevalence of diabetic retinopathy. For the treatment, management, and prevention of retinopathy, special attention is required for patients with other comorbidities.

The study reported that fasting blood glucose, serum total cholesterol, serum triglyceride, and HbA1c are independent risk factors for diabetic retinopathy. Metabolic abnormalities have a significant role in the prevalence of diabetic retinopathy because they may worsen the chronic complications of diabetes mellitus.

The study reported that IOP, cup–disc ratio, and disc asymmetry including the cup–disc ratio are not associated with diabetic retinopathy. Unlike comorbidities and metabolic syndrome, the small amount of increase in IOP would not lead to diabetic retinopathy.

There are several limitations of the study which as a lack of random sampling in the cross-sectional study. However, the study reported glaucoma, age-related macular degeneration, and other pathogenesis for ocular fundus diseases but did not evaluate the risk factors for the same.

The intra-and inter-rater agreements are required to perform between ophthalmologists for image analysis of fundus photographs but the study did not perform agreements. The current study reported only a few patients with myopia but a census population-based survey estimated the prevalence of myopia to be very high in young people in Eastern China. The patients enrolled in the current study are older than a population-based survey. The current study reported a significant number of patients with glaucoma but a recent meta-analysis found the prevalence of glaucoma in China to be very low, considering the entire large population. Serial measurement of IOP, optic nerve, and visual fields especially in the early stage of the disease, shows a close relationship between Diabetes mellitus and retinopathy. As a result, the current study overestimated glaucoma in the population. The current study did not consider the age of the patient when diagnosing age-related macular degeneration. Relatively young patients can have these findings as a result of an alternative etiology such as pattern dystrophy or myopic maculopathy. Additionally, the study did not differentiate between wet and dry age-related macular degeneration. It also did not differentiate between proliferative and non-proliferative retinopathy.

Conclusions

Diabetic retinopathy is the most common ocular fundus disease in diabetic patients. Also, age, sex, hypertension, duration of diabetes, diabetic neuropathy, diabetic nephropathy, diabetic foot ulcer, foot amputation, fasting blood glucose, serum total cholesterol, serum triglyceride, and HbA1c are independent risk factors for diabetic retinopathy.

Footnotes

Abbreviations: BMI = body mass index, HbA1c = glycated hemoglobin, IOP = intraocular pressure, STROBE=the study reporting adheres to the strengthening of the reporting of observational studies in epidemiology.

How to cite this article: Yin L, Zhang D, Ren Q, Su X, Sun Z. Prevalence and risk factors of diabetic retinopathy in diabetic patients: A community-based cross-sectional study. Medicine. 2020;99:9(e19236).

The data sets used and analyzed during the current study are available from the corresponding author upon reasonable request.

The research did not receive any specific financial motivation from the government of PR China, non-government, or non-profitable sectors to perform research.

The authors have no conflicts of interest to disclose.

References

AlEssa, H., Bhupathiraju, S., Malik, V., Wedick, N., Campos, H., Rosner, B., Willett, W., & Hu, F. B. (2015). Abstract 20: Carbohydrate Quality, Measured Using Multiple Carbohydrate Quality Metrics, is Negatively Associated with Risk of Type 2 Diabetes in US Women. Circulation, 131(suppl_1). https://doi.org/10.1161/CIRC.131.SUPPL_1.20

Cardiovascular diseases (CVDs). (n.d.). Retrieved September 9, 2022, from

https://www.who.int/news-room/fact-sheets/detail/cardiovascular-diseases- (cvds)

de Koning, L., Malik, V. S., Rimm, E. B., Willett, W. C., & Hu, F. B. (2011). Sugar-sweetened and artificially sweetened beverage consumption and risk of type 2 diabetes in men. The American Journal of Clinical Nutrition, 93(6), 1321–1327. https://doi.org/10.3945/AJCN.110.007922

de Munter, J. S. L., Hu, F. B., Spiegelman, D., Franz, M., & van Dam, R. M. (2007). Whole grain, bran, and germ intake and risk of type 2 diabetes: A prospective cohort study and systematic review. PLoS Medicine, 4(8),1385–1395.https://doi.org/10.1371/JOURNAL.PMED.0040261

Djoussé, L., Biggs, M. L., Mukamal, K. J., & Siscovick, D. S. (2007). Alcohol consumption and type 2 diabetes among older adults: The cardiovascular health study. Obesity, 15(7), 1758–1765. https://doi.org/10.1038/OBY.2007.209

Florez, J. C., Jablonski, K. A., Bayley, N., Pollin, T. I., de Bakker, P. I. W., Shuldiner, A. R., Knowler, W. C., Nathan, D. M., & Altshuler, D. (2006). TCF7L2 Polymorphisms and Progression to Diabetes in the Diabetes Prevention Program. In n engl j med (Vol. 355). www.nejm.org

High Blood Pressure Symptoms and Causes | cdc.gov. (n.d.). Retrieved August 13, 2022, from https://www.cdc.gov/bloodpressure/about.htm

Malik, V. S., Popkin, B. M., Bray, G. A., Després, J. P., & Hu, F. B. (2010). Sugar-sweetened beverages, obesity, type 2 diabetes mellitus, and cardiovascular disease risk. Circulation, 121(11), 1356–1364. https://doi.org/10.1161/CIRCULATIONAHA.109.876185

Meigs, J. B., Shrader, P., Sullivan, L. M., McAteer, J. B., Fox, C. S., Dupuis, J., Manning, A.

K., Florez, J. C., Wilson, P. W., D, R. B., Adrienne Cupples, L., & Meigs, J. (2008). Genotype Score in Addition to Common Risk Factors for Prediction of Type 2 Diabetes Abstract. In N Engl J Med (Vol. 359). www.nejm.org

Mozaffarian, D., Katan, M. B., Ascherio, A., Stampfer, M. J., & Willett, W. C. (2006). Trans Fatty Acids and Cardiovascular Disease. New England Journal of Medicine, 354(15), 1601–1613. https://doi.org/10.1056/NEJMRA054035

Rank, F., Nn, J. O. A., Anson, E. M., Eir, M., Tampfer, J. S., Raham, G., Olditz, C., Olomon,

A. G. S., Alter, W., & Illett, C. W. (2001). The New Eng land Journal of Medicine DIET, LIFESTYLE, AND THE RISK OF TYPE 2 DIABETES MELLITUS IN WOMEN ABSTRACT. N Engl J Med, 345(11). www.nejm.org

Risérus, U., Willett, W. C., & Hu, F. B. (2009). Dietary fats and prevention of type 2 diabetes.

Progress in Lipid Research, 48(1), 44–51. https://doi.org/10.1016/j.plipres.2008.10.002

Tanasescu, M., Leitzmann, M. F., Rimm, E. B., & Hu, F. B. (2003). Physical activity in relation to cardiovascular disease and total mortality among men with type 2 diabetes.

Circulation, 107(19), 2435–2439. https://doi.org/10.1161/01.CIR.0000066906.11109.1F

Vartanian, L. R., Schwartz, M. B., & Brownell, K. D. (2007). Effects of soft drink consumption on nutrition and health: A systematic review and meta-analysis. American Journal of Public Health, 97(4), 667–675. https://doi.org/10.2105/AJPH.2005.083782

What Is Cancer? - NCI. (n.d.). Retrieved September 17, 2022, from https://www.cancer.gov/about-cancer/understanding/what-is-cancer

Wood, S., Harrison, S. E., Judd, N., Bellis, M. A., Hughes, K., & Jones, A. (2021). The impact of behavioral risk factors on communicable diseases: a systematic review of reviews. BMC Public Health, 21(1), 1– 16. https://doi.org/10.1186/S12889-021-12148-Y/PEER-REVIEW

AlEssa, H., Bhupathiraju, S., Malik, V., Wedick, N., Campos, H., Rosner, B., Willett, W., & Hu, F. B. (2015). Abstract 20: Carbohydrate Quality, Measured Using Multiple Carbohydrate Quality Metrics, is Negatively Associated with Risk of Type 2 Diabetes in US Women. Circulation, 131(suppl_1). https://doi.org/10.1161/CIRC.131.SUPPL_1.20

Cardiovascular diseases (CVDs). (n.d.). Retrieved September 9, 2022, from https://www.who.int/news-room/fact-sheets/detail/cardiovascular-diseases- (cvds)

de Koning, L., Malik, V. S., Rimm, E. B., Willett, W. C., & Hu, F. B. (2011). Sugar-sweetened and artificially sweetened beverage consumption and risk of type 2 diabetes in men. The American Journal of Clinical Nutrition, 93(6), 1321–1327. https://doi.org/10.3945/AJCN.110.007922

de Munter, J. S. L., Hu, F. B., Spiegelman, D., Franz, M., & van Dam, R. M. (2007). Whole grain, bran, and germ intake and risk of type 2 diabetes: A prospective cohort study and systematic review. PLoS Medicine, 4(8),1385–1395. https://doi.org/10.1371/JOURNAL.PMED.0040261

Djoussé, L., Biggs, M. L., Mukamal, K. J., & Siscovick, D. S. (2007). Alcohol consumption and type 2 diabetes among older adults: The cardiovascular health study. Obesity, 15(7), 1758–1765. https://doi.org/10.1038/OBY.2007.209

Florez, J. C., Jablonski, K. A., Bayley, N., Pollin, T. I., de Bakker, P. I. W., Shuldiner, A. R., Knowler, W. C., Nathan, D. M., & Altshuler, D. (2006). TCF7L2 Polymorphisms and Progression to Diabetes in the Diabetes Prevention Program. In n engl j med (Vol. 355). www.nejm.org

High Blood Pressure Symptoms and Causes | cdc.gov. (n.d.). Retrieved August 13, 2022, from https://www.cdc.gov/bloodpressure/about. htm

Malik, V. S., Popkin, B. M., Bray, G. A., Després, J. P., & Hu, F. B. (2010). Sugar-sweetened beverages, obesity, type 2 diabetes mellitus, and cardiovascular disease risk. Circulation, 121(11), 1356–1364. https://doi.org /10.1161/CIRCULATIONAHA.109.876185

Meigs, J. B., Shrader, P., Sullivan, L. M., McAteer, J. B., Fox, C. S., Dupuis, J., Manning, A.

K., Florez, J. C., Wilson, P. W., D, R. B., Adrienne Cupples, L., & Meigs, J. (2008). Genotype Score in Addition to Common Risk Factors for Prediction of Type 2 Diabetes A bs tr ac t. In N Engl J Med (Vol. 359). www.nejm.org

Mozaffarian, D., Katan, M. B., Ascherio, A., Stampfer, M. J., & Willett, W. C. (2006). Trans Fatty Acids and Cardiovascular Disease. New England Journal of Medicine, 354(15), 1601–1613. https://doi.org /10.1056/NEJMRA054035

Rank, F., Nn, J. O. A., Anson, E. M., Eir, M., Tampfer, J. S., Raham, G., Olditz, C., Olomon,

A. G. S., Alter, W., & Ilett, C. W. (2001). The New England Journal of Medicine DIET, LIFESTYLE, AND THE RISK OF TYPE 2 DIABETES MELLITUS IN WOMEN ABSTRACT. N Engl J Med, 345(11). www.nejm.org Risérus, U., Willett, W. C., & Hu, F. B. (2009).Dietary fats and prevention of type 2 diabetes.

Progress in Lipid Research, 48(1), 44–51. https://doi.org/10.1016/j.plipres.2008.10.002 Tanasescu, M., Leitzmann, M. F., Rimm, E. B., & Hu, F. B. (2003). Physical activity in relation to cardiovascular disease and total mortality among men with type 2 diabetes. Circulation, 107(19), 2435–2439. https://doi.org /10.1161/01.CIR.0000066906.11109.1F

Vartanian, L. R., Schwartz, M. B., & Brownell, K. D. (2007). Effects of soft drink consumption on nutrition and health: A systematic review and meta-analysis. American Journal of Public Health, 97(4), 667–675.

https://doi.org/10.2105/AJPH.2005.083782 What Is Cancer? - NCI. (n.d.). Retrieved September 17, 2022, from

https://www.cancer.gov/about-cancer/understanding/what-is-cancer

Wood, S., Harrison, S. E., Judd, N., Bellis, M. A., Hughes, K., & Jones, A. (2021). The impact of behavioral risk factors on communicable diseases: a systematic review of reviews. BMC Public Health, 21(1), 1–16.

https://doi.org/10.1186/S12889-021- 12148-Y/PEERREVIEW

MaRC.Epidemiology of diabetes and diabetic complications in China. Diabetologia 2018;61:1249–60. [PubMed] [Google Scholar]

Xue, WangL, HeJ, et al. PrevalenceandcontrolofdiabetesinChinese adults. JAMA 2013;310:948–59. [PubMed] [Google Scholar]

Liu Z, Fu C, Wang W, et al. Prevalence of chronic complications of type 2 diabetes mellitus in an outpatients-across-sectional hospital-based survey in urban China. Health Qual Life Outcomes 2010;8:1–9. [PMC free article] [PubMed] [Google Scholar]

Yang L, Shao J, Bian Y, et al. Prevalence of type 2 diabetes mellitus among inland residents in China (2000-2014): a meta-analysis. JDiabetes Investig 2016;7:845–52. [PMC free article] [PubMed] [Google Scholar]

Yang W, Lu J, Weng J, et al. Prevalence of diabetes among men and women in China. N Engl J Med 2010;362:1090–101. [PubMed] [Google Scholar]

Liu L, Geng J, Wu J, et al. Prevalence of ocular fundus pathology with type 2 diabetesina Chinese urban community as assessed by tele screening.BMJ Open 2014;3:1–7. [PMCfreearticle] [PubMed] [GoogleScholar]

Choi JK, Lym YL, Moon JW, et al. Diabetes mellitus and early age-related macular degeneration.ArchOphthalmol 2011;129:196– 9.[PubMed][GoogleScholar] Tan GS, Wong TY, Fong CW, et al. Singapore Malay Eye Study. Diabetes, metabolic abnormalities, and glaucoma.Arch Ophthalmol 2009;127:1354–61. [PubMed] [GoogleScholar]

Tangy, WangX, WangJ, et al. Prevalence and causes of visual impairment in Chineseadultpopulation:theTaizhoueyestudy.Ophthalmology 2015;122:1 480– 8.[PubMed][GoogleScholar]

Zhang G, Chen H, Chen W, et al. Prevalence and risk factors for diabetic retinopathy in China: a multi-hospital-based cross-sectional study.Br J Ophthalmol 2017;101:1591–5. [PMC free article] [PubMed] [Google Scholar]

Sapkota R, Chen Z, Zheng D, et al. The profile of sight-threatening diabetic retinopathy in patients attending a specialist eye clinic in Hangzhou.China BMJ Open Ophthalmol 2019;4:1–6. [PMC free article] [PubMed] [Google Scholar]

Walton OB, 4th, Garoon RB, Weng CY, et al. Evaluation of automated tele retinal screening program for diabetic retinopathy. JAMA Ophthalmol 2016;134:204–9. [PubMed] [GoogleScholar]

Villena JE, Yoshiyama CA, Sanchez JE, et al. Prevalence of diabetic retinopathy in Peruvian patients with type 2 diabetes: results of a hospital-based retinal telescreens program.Rev Panam Salud Publica 2011;30:408–14. [PubMed] [Google Scholar] von Elm E, Altman DG, Egger M, et al. The strengthening of the reporting of observational studies in epidemiology (STROBE) statement: guidelines for reporting observational studies.Int J Surg 2014;12:1495–9.[PubMed][GoogleScholar]

Willekens K, Bataille S, Sarens I, et al. Funduscopic versus HRT III confocal scanner vertical cup-disc ratio assessment in normal tension and primary open angle glaucoma (The Leuven Eye Study).Ophthalmic Res2017;57:100–6. [PubMed] [GoogleScholar]

Zheng Y, Wong TY, Cheung CY, et al. Influence of diabetes and diabetic retinopathy on the performance of Heidelberg retina tomography II for diagnosis of glaucoma. Invest Ophthalmol Vis Sci 2010;51:5519– 24.[PubMed][GoogleScholar]

Pang C, Jia L, Hou X, et al. The significance of screening for microvascular diseases in Chinese community-based subjects with various metabolic abnormalities.PLoSOne2014;9:1–6.[PMCfreearticle][PubMed][Google Scholar]

Liu, Yue, Wu J, et al. Prevalence and risk factors of retinopathy in patients with or without metabolic syndrome: a population-based study in Shenyang.BMJ Open 2015;5:1–7. [PMC freearticle] [PubMed] [Google Scholar]

Thapa R, Bajimaya S, Bouman R, et al. Intra- and inter-rater agreement between an ophthalmologist and mid-level ophthalmic personnel to diagnose retinal diseases based on fundus photographs at a primary eye center in Nepal: the Bhaktapur RetinaStudy.BMCOphthalmol 2016;16:1–6.[PMCfreearticle] [PubMed] [Google Scholar]

Chen M, Wu A, Zhang L, et al.The increasing prevalence of myopia and high myopia among high school students in Fenghua city, eastern China: a 15-year population-based survey.

BMCOphthalmol 2018;18:1– 0. [PMC freearticle] [PubMed] [GoogleScholar]

Song P, Wang J, Buccan K, et al. National and subnational prevalence and burden of glaucoma main China: a systematic analysis.JGlobHealth2017;7:114–31.[PMCfreearticle][PubMed][GoogleScholar]

Printed in Dunstable, United Kingdom

65310526R00090